CHAPTER LEADER'S GUIDE TO

Medical Staff

Practical Insight on
Joint Commission Standards

⊢CPro

Matt Phillion, Editor
Michael Briddon, Executive Editor
Emily Sheahan, Group Publisher
Susan Darbyshire, Cover Designer

Mike Mirabello, Senior Graphic Artist
Karin Holmes, Copyeditor
Matt Sharpe, Production Supervisor
Jean St. Pierre, Senior Director of Operations

Advice given is general. Readers should consult professional counsel for specific legal, ethical, or clinical questions. Arrangements can be made for quantity discounts. For more information, contact

HCPro, Inc.
75 Sylvan Street, Suite A-101
Danvers, MA 01923
Telephone: 800/650-6787 or 781/639-1872
Fax: 800/639-8511
E-mail: *customerservice@hcpro.com*

Visit HCPro online at: *www.hcpro.com* and *www.hcmarketplace.com*

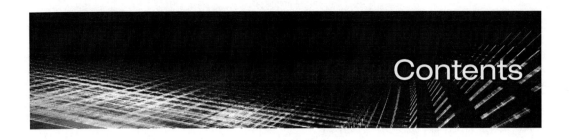

Contents

CONTENTS

CONTENTS

About the Author

Kathy Matzka, CPMSM, CPCS

Kathy Matzka, CPMSM, CPCS, is a speaker, consultant, and writer with over 20 years of experience in credentialing, privileging, and medical staff services. She holds certification by the National Association Medical Staff Services (NAMSS) in both Medical Staff Management and Provider Credentialing. She worked for 13 years as a hospital medical staff coordinator before venturing out on her own as a consultant, writer, and speaker.

Kathy has authored a number of books related to medical staff services including both the fifth and sixth editions of the *Compliance Guide to Joint Commission Medical Staff Standards*, and *The Medical Staff Meeting Companion Tools and Techniques for Effective Presentations*. For the past eight years, she has been the contributing editor for the credentialing industry's premier credentialing publication, *The Credentials Verification Desk Reference,* and its companion website *The Credentialing and Privileging Desktop Reference.*

She has performed extensive work with NAMSS' Library Team developing and editing educational materials related to the field including *CPCS Certification Exam Preparatory Course, NAMSS Core Curriculum, CPMSM and CPCS Professional Development Workshops,* and *Independent Study Programs.* These programs are essential educational tools for both new and seasoned medical services professionals. She also serves as a speaker and instructor for NAMSS.

Kathy shares her expertise by serving on the editorial advisory boards for three publications: *Briefings on Credentialing, Credentialing and Peer Review Legal Insider,* and *Advisor for Medical and Professional Staff Services.*

Kathy is a highly regarded industry speaker, and in this role has developed and presented numerous programs for professional associations, hospitals, and hospital associations on a wide range of topics including provider credentialing and privileging, medical staff meeting management, peer review, negligent credentialing, provider competency, and accreditation standards.

In her spare time, Kathy takes pleasure in spending time with her family, listening to music, singing with her church worship team, traveling, hiking, fishing, and other outdoor activities.

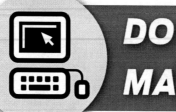

DOWNLOAD YOUR MATERIALS NOW

Sample tools and documents from this book, including a special PowerPoint® presentation to help readers communicate these materials with their staff, are available online at the website listed below. This is an additional service provided by HCPro, Inc., and the authors of our *Chapter Leader's Guide* series.

www.hcpro.com/downloads/9136

Thank you for purchasing this product!

HCPro

PART 1

Medical Staff Standard: The High-Level Overview

How Does This Chapter Affect the Organization as a Whole?

The standards contained in the Medical Staff chapter focus mainly on governance and organization of the medical staff, credentialing and privileging licensed independent practitioners, and overseeing the clinical activities of those practitioners.

The quality of the care provided by the medical staff is a huge factor in the public's view of the hospital. The hospital can be providing services at a scale that exceeds the standard of care, but if the medical staff is not performing to the standard of care, it will make the services provided by the hospital appear to be below standard. Likewise, the perceived performance of the hospital also reflects on the overall view of care provided in the community. As such, compliance with the medical staff standards can have an impact on the public's perception of the entire hospital and even the surrounding community.

What Is Its Impact on Leadership/Administration?

It is essential that the medical staff's functions are well supported and monitored continuously by the hospital. Hospital administration and leadership must be aware of the skill set and education necessary to support the medical staff's functions.

Since medical staff leadership skills are not included in the training provided in medical school and postgraduate programs, these skills must be learned, and it typically falls to the hospital to equip medical staff leaders for their jobs. In fact, The Joint Commission's leadership standards require that medical staff leaders have the knowledge necessary to carry out their roles in the hospital and that the governing body provides access to information and training in areas where additional skills or expertise are necessary.

Most of the hospital's responsibilities with regard to support of the medical staff's functions are carried out by the medical services professional (MSP), who is a part of the hospital's administrative team. The medical staff office (MSO) must be adequately staffed with properly educated and trained personnel to effectively and efficiently meet the needs of the medical staff. Adequate space is needed for MSPs to work, to have a secure area in which to house practitioner credentials files, peer review documents, minute books, etc. MSPs also must be supplied with adequate computer hardware/software and office equipment. The issue of staffing the MSO is significant since credentialing and privileging are essential functions and carry a considerable amount of risk to both patient safety and the hospital if not performed to the generally recognized standard. This is evidenced by the increasing number of negligent credentialing lawsuits.

The job of the MSP requires maintaining a certain level of expertise and knowledge. In order for this to happen, it is essential that ongoing education be supported by the hospital.

In addition, the leadership standards assign responsibility to the governing body for making sure that medical staff leaders have the appropriate level of access to information as well as sufficient training to perform their jobs. Since medical staff leadership duties are not taught in medical school or postgraduate training programs, the hospital must assume the job of training its medical staff leaders.

Who Owns the Requirements of This Chapter?

At one time, The Joint Commission's medical staff standards were neatly contained in one chapter, making it easy to determine what aspects of the survey pertained to the medical staff. Now, standards relating to the medical staff are interspersed throughout almost all sections of the standards.

The Joint Commission has entitled the chapter "Medical Staff" and the medical staff is assigned responsibility for most of the functions. Although the medical staff does fulfill important functions, particularly in the areas of quality assessment, performance improvement, and peer review, in reality, the bulk of the work required to accomplish these functions falls to the hospital. Without the support of medical staff services and quality professionals, hospital administrators, department managers, and the governing body, it would be very difficult, if not impossible, for the medical staff to comply with the accreditation standards.

Responsibility for many standards is assigned to the hospital. This includes determining necessary resources to support privilege requests, collection of credentialing information, performing primary source verification, establishing credentialing criteria, development of procedures for processing applications, determining whether sufficient information is available to make a privileging decision, collecting/investigating/addressing clinical practice concerns, and performing educational activities.

The medical services professional (MSP)

The MSP is typically the person responsible for management of all medical staff processes. Specific activities include:

- Ensuring that the application and reapplication process are completed within the required time period and per bylaws and policies

- Prescreening to ensure that the applicant meets the medical staff's minimum criteria for appointment and clinical privileges

- Conducting primary source verification of all credentials

- Assembling all verified information and preparing the applicant's credentials file for review by the credentials committee, the medical staff department chief, and the medical executive committee (MEC)

- Notifying appropriate individuals regarding privileging actions

- Maintaining an ongoing tickler system for reappointment of staff members

- Collecting and verifying on an ongoing basis credentials that expire

- Orientating new medical staff members and leaders

- Providing coordination and support for meetings

- Researching and accumulating documentation necessary to develop privileging criteria

- Ensuring that bylaws are up-to-date

- Serving as the organization's expert with respect to accreditation standards and regulations regarding the medical staff

The quality staff's role

The quality staff supports and coordinates the medical staff's quality assessment, performance improvement, focused and ongoing professional practice evaluation, and the peer review processes. They do this through the accumulation, analysis, and reporting of data to the medical staff. The medical staff then uses these data to make recommendations to improve patient care and in their decisions to approve, limit, or discontinue clinical privileges. The quality staff also coordinates chart reviews as part of the peer review process. This may include initial screening of charts using criteria approved by the medical staff.

The medical staff's role

The medical staff's role varies depending on the size and structure of the medical staff. A large hospital's medical staff may have a number of departments and committees performing required functions. In small hospitals, the medical staff as a whole may perform these functions.

The following are the common medical staff roles:

- *The department chair's role:* The department chair must be able to look at the big picture and see how his or her department functions with respect to the entire healthcare organization. He or she reviews credentials, applications, verifications, and all supporting information and makes a recommendation to the credentials committee/MEC regarding the applicant's qualifications and competency to perform the privileges requested. There are also a number of responsibilities spelled out in the standards, which are addressed in Part 2.

- *The credentials committee chair's role:* Although The Joint Commission does not require a credentials committee, many hospitals utilize such a committee. The credentials committee chair oversees the hospital's credentialing program and is responsible for making sure all credentialing activities comply with the hospital's credentialing policies, accreditation standards, and all other applicable laws and regulations. The credentials committee is responsible for reviewing each completed credentials file, reviewing the department chair's recommendations, and making recommendations to the MEC regarding staff appointment, reappointment, and clinical privileges. The credentials committee may also interview applicants. (See this book's resource download page for a sample PowerPoint® presentation that can be used for orientating credentials committee members.)

- *The medical executive committee's role:* The MEC receives the recommendations of the department chair and credentials committee. It is responsible for submitting a recommendation to the hospital's governing body regarding appointment, reappointment, and clinical privileges. The MEC acts for the medical staff in between meetings. There are also a number of responsibilities spelled out in the standards, which are addressed in Part 2.

The chief executive officer's role

The CEO is responsible for the day-to-day operations of the hospital. The CEO is typically responsible for ensuring that medical staff leaders and hospital staff are trained appropriately regarding their responsibilities under Joint Commission standards and have adequate resources to complete their functions. He or she attends the MEC meetings as an ex officio member. The CEO is responsible for granting temporary privileges on recommendation of the medical staff president. Typically, the CEO coordinates the flow of information between the medical staff and governing body.

The hospital governing body's role

The governing body considers the recommendations of the medical staff and makes the final decision regarding appointment, reappointment, and granting privileges. It also approves and complies with medical staff bylaws. The governing body is the final authority in these decisions.

Key players by standard

The following outline breaks down the individual sections of the standards and shows the key players in compliance with each standard. (Note: This will vary depending on the hospital structure and the roles and assigned responsibilities of individual employees.) This document is also available on the website. You may customize it to your facility's needs.

1.1 Hospital Medical Staff (MS) Standards and Key Players Outline

Standard and Element of Performance	Medical Staff	Medical Staff Leaders	MEC	Medical Services Professional	Quality Professional	CEO	Governing Body	Other
I. Medical Staff bylaws								
A. Bylaws (MS.01.01.01)	X	X	X	X		X	X	Hospital and/or medical staff legal counsel
B. No Unilateral Amendment (MS.01.01.03)	X	X	X				X	
II. Structure and Role of Medical Staff Executive Committee (MS.02.01.01)	X	X	X	X		X		
III. Medical Staff Role in Oversight of Care, Treatment, and Services								
A. Oversight of Quality of Care (MS.03.01.01)	X	X	X	X	X		X	• HIM director • Emergency department manager • Radiology dept. manager • Nuclear services department manager
B. Management and Coordination of Care (MS.03.01.03)	X	X		X				Educator for pain management
IV. Medical Staff Role in Graduate Education Programs (MS.04.01.01)	X	X	X	X	X	X	X	• GME program supervisors and director • GME committee • Community or local hospital participating in program

1.1 — Hospital Medical Staff (MS) Standards and Key Players Outline *(cont.)*

Standard and Element of Performance	Medical Staff	Medical Staff Leaders	MEC	Medical Services Professional	Quality Professional	CEO	Governing Body	Other
V. Medical Staff Role in Performance Improvement								
A. Role in Performance Improvement Activities (MS.05.01.01)	X	X	X	X	X	X	X	• Pharmacy director • Blood bank director • Surgical services director • Pathology director • Hospital safety director • Nurse manager
B. Participation in Performance Improvement Activities (MS.05.01.03)	X	X	X	X	X	X	X	• Patient educator • Hospital personnel involved with care of patient • HIM director
VI. Credentialing								
A. Determining Resource Availability (MS.06.01.01)		X	X	X		X	X	Department managers for services to be evaluated
B. Collecting Credentialing Information (MS.06.01.03)	X	X	X	X		X	X	• Supervising radiologist • Hospital staff involved with verifying identity of practitioner • CVO

 9

1.1 Hospital Medical Staff (MS) Standards and Key Players Outline *(cont.)*

Standard and Element of Performance	Medical Staff	Medical Staff Leaders	MEC	Medical Services Professional	Quality Professional	CEO	Governing Body	Other
VII. Privileging								
A. Privileging Decision Process (MS.06.01.05)	X	X	X	X	X	X	X	
B. Review and Analysis of Information (MS.06.01.07)	X	X	X	X		X	X	
C. Communicating Decision (MS.06.01.09)	X	X	X	X		X	X	• Hospital staff who receive information concerning privileging decisions • Hospital legal consul (adverse decisions)
D. Expedited Privileging Process (MS.06.01.11)	X	X		X		X	X	Administrative support staff for CEO/governing body
E. Temporary Privileges (MS.06.01.13)	X	X		X		X		
VIII. Appointment to Medical Staff								
A. Recommending Appointment (MS.07.01.01)	X	X	X	X		X	X	
B. Peer Recommendations (MS.07.01.03)	X	X	X	X				
IX. Evaluation of Practitioners								
A. Focused Professional Practice Evaluation (MS.08.01.01)	X	X	X	X	X	X		

1.1 Hospital Medical Staff (MS) Standards and Key Players Outline *(cont.)*

Standard and Element of Performance	Medical Staff	Medical Staff Leaders	MEC	Medical Services Professional	Quality Professional	CEO	Governing Body	Other
B. Ongoing Professional Practice Evaluation (MS.08.01.03)	X	X	X	X	X	X	X	• Individual medical staff departments • Pharmacy director • Blood bank director • Surgical services director • Pathology director • Hospital safety director • Nurse managers • Infection control manager
X. Acting on Reported Concerns About a Practitioner (MS.09.01.01)	X	X	X	X	X	X	X	Hospital staff and/or patients who report concerns
XI. Fair Hearing and Appeal Process (MS.10.01.01)	X	X	X	X	X	X	X	Hospital and/or medical staff legal consul
XII. Licensed Independent Practitioner Health (MS.11.01.01)	X	X	X	X		X	X	Hospital and/or medical staff legal consul
XIII. Continuing Medical Education (MS.12.01.01)	X	X		X	X			Hospital education coordinator
XIV. Telemedicine								
A. Credentialing and Privileging of Licensed Independent Practitioners (MS.13.01.01)	X	X	X	X	X	X	X	Distant site staff
B. Recommending Clinical Services to Be Provided (MS.13.01.03)	X	X	X	X		X	X	Distant site staff

Medical Staff Standards: The Mid-Level View

How Do You Communicate These Standards to Those Who Need It?

What is the impact of these standards on caregivers/nurses/staff? What do they mean for physicians?

As noted in the previous chapter, the medical staff standards are not just for the medical staff. Many standards reflect organizational responsibility. In some cases, there may be responsibilities that fall under the job duties of a hospital employee and that staff member may not even know about them. For example, MS.03.01.03, EP 2 requires that the hospital educate all licensed independent practitioners (LIP) regarding assessing and managing pain. The hospital may have a nursing educator who is responsible for educating hospital staff regarding pain management but may not realize that this training must be extended to nonemployee LIPs. There are responsibilities of the governing body regarding the option for expedited credentialing that board members may not be aware of if they do not read the Medical Staff chapter.

Hospital staff

The Hospital Medical Staff (MS) Standards and Key Players Outline chart included in Part 1 and on this book's downloadable resource Web page can be used to quickly identify those who need to be involved in assessing organizational compliance and implementing standards requirements. Using this chart, identify who is responsible for the element of performance. Meet with each of these staff members and make sure he or she understands the requirements and evaluate what is being done to comply.

The following are areas in which there are MS standards that apply to the hospital staff:

- **MS.04.01.01:** The medical staff and hospital staff must be provided with written descriptions of the roles, responsibilities, and patient care activities of graduate medical education program participants. This standard contains the (D) icon, which requires documentation to determine compliance.

- **MS.11.01.01:** The medical staff must have a process to identify and manage health matters of LIPs. This process must be separate from the disciplinary action process and must include education of LIPs and organization staff regarding recognizing illness and impairment issues specific to LIPs. This EP requires specific training regarding recognizing and dealing with impairment, including defining "at-risk" behaviors. Educate hospital staff as well as medical staff about the policy because they need to know what constitutes impaired/disruptive behavior and when and how to report an incident. Your state medical society may be able to help with this training and education.

Credentials committee

If the organization utilizes a credentials committee, orientation of its members is essential. The presentation posted to this book's download page includes typical responsibilities of the credentials committee and can be customized to include information about meeting dates, how credentials files are set up, and key contact information. Schedule ongoing educational activities for members of the credentials committee to keep them informed of any changes in accreditation standards and regulatory requirements and to address any questions they might have regarding their role and responsibilities. The website also contains a customizable slide presentation on credentialing and privileging basics that can be used for orienting members regarding these issues.

Department chair

MS standards include a comprehensive list of the roles and responsibilities of the department chair. Although hospital employees may carry out some administrative functions, The Joint Commission assigns some responsibilities to the department chair, so the chair needs to be aware of these responsibilities. Schedule an appointment with each department chair to review these requirements. Include the hospital employee in charge of each department that falls under the chair's direction. This is particularly important for department chairs of hospital-based services, such as radiology, emergency medicine, and anesthesiology, whose position may involve a contractual arrangement that includes oversight of staff and services provided by the department. Areas of responsibility required by MS standards are:

- Clinically related activities of the department.

- Administratively related activities of the department. (This standard doesn't apply if the hospital is providing administrative support. For instance, if the medical staff has an emergency medicine department and the hospital employs a manager to oversee the administrative functions of the emergency department, the department chair would not be held to this standard.)

- Continuing observation of the professional performance of LIPs in the department.

- Making recommendations to the medical staff regarding the criteria for clinical privileges within the department.

- Making recommendations regarding each department member's clinical privileges.

- Evaluating and making recommendations regarding any off-site sources of patient care, treatment, and services that are not provided by the department or the organization. (For example, if the hospital does not have an MRI unit, the medical staff would evaluate and make recommendations regarding any off-site services.)

- Integrating the department into the primary functions of the organization and coordinating and integrating interdepartmental and intradepartmental services. These standards require the department chair to look at the big picture and how his or her department functions with respect to the entire healthcare organization.

- Developing and implementing policies and procedures that guide the department and support the provision of care, treatment, and services.

- Recommending an adequate number of qualified and competent persons to provide care, treatment, and services. This standard is particularly important for medical staff departments that support a hospital department, such as radiology, emergency services, pathology, etc.

- Determining qualifications and competency for non-LIP departmental personnel providing patient care, treatment, or services.

- Ongoing assessment and improvement of the quality of patient care, treatment, and services.

- Maintaining quality control programs.

- Orienting and providing continuing education of all persons in the department or service.

- Recommending space and other needed departmental resources.

Medical executive committee

Joint Commission standards require that a medical executive committee (MEC) be formed. The individual EPs describe the functions, composition, and responsibilities of the MEC and what needs to be documented in the medical staff bylaws. The Joint Commission does not attempt to tell hospitals what the makeup of the MEC should be, but it does require that all medical staff members and the hospital CEO be allowed to participate. Your hospital's medical staff is free to define the structure. It may be composed of elected or appointed department directors or it may be a body of elected members. In a hospital with a small medical staff, the medical staff as a whole may serve as the executive committee. In this case, the medical staff is known as a "committee of the whole." Joint Commission standards assign the following duties to the MEC, which should be included in the medical staff bylaws:

- In intervals between medical staff meetings, the MEC acts on behalf of the medical staff.

- Having a mechanism for recommending terminations of medical staff membership.

- When there is a question about the ability to perform the privileges granted for a practitioner privileged through the medical staff process, the MEC must request an evaluation of that practitioner. The MEC should evaluate the results of the medical staff performance improvement (PI) activities. If these activities identify a problem provider or a provider who is functioning below the acceptable level of care, the MEC must take action. This action should be documented in the minutes of the MEC meeting or in an attached addendum to those minutes.

- Make recommendations to the governing body regarding the structure of the medical staff.

- Make recommendations to the governing body regarding the process for reviewing credentials and delineating privileges.

- Make recommendations to the governing body regarding delineating privileges for all practitioners who are privileged through the medical staff process. (This includes practitioners such as advanced practice nurses and physician assistants who are granted privileges without being granted medical staff appointment.)

- Make recommendations to the governing body regarding the MEC's authority to review and act on the reports of medical staff committees, departments, and other groups or committees who are assigned a specific function. Medical staff departments, standing committees, and ad hoc committees make their recommendations to the MEC, which then takes action or makes recommendations to the governing body.

Discuss each of these responsibilities at a meeting of the MEC. Make sure members know the processes utilized for each of these functions. The website contains a customizable slide presentation on credentialing and privileging basics that can be used for orienting MEC members regarding these issues.

Things to evaluate include:

- Review medical staff bylaws to make sure all required elements are contained.

- Compare a listing of the actual committee members with the requirements in the bylaws to determine whether they are consistent. The structure and function of the MEC must conform to what is documented in the medical staff bylaws.

- Review committee attendance. The hospital's CEO or designee should be attending each MEC meeting on an ex officio basis, with or without a vote. Ex officio means by virtue of one's office. The term refers to the practice that allows someone to participate on a committee because of the position he or she holds. Generally, ex officio members do not vote, but this decision is up to the organization.

- Review bylaws to be sure that, regardless of specialty, all medical staff members are eligible for membership on the MEC. If your medical staff grants medical staff membership to advanced practice nurses or other LIPs, then these categories of practitioners should be eligible for MEC membership. If you have revised your bylaws to allow these providers to become medical staff members, check your bylaws language regarding the MEC to make sure it allows these practitioners to participate in this committee.

- Check to be sure that the majority of voting members of the MEC are fully licensed physicians who are *actively* practicing in the hospital. This is particularly important if the hospital has recently implemented a hospitalist program, as there may be committee members who were actively practicing in the hospital when they were appointed to the MEC and have subsequently turned over their inpatient practice to a hospitalist.

Governing body

Because the governing body or board is the ultimate authority in the hospital and is responsible for granting medical staff appointment and clinical privileges, it is essential that the board understand the credentialing and privileging processes and that board members are aware of the MS standards that reflect these responsibilities. The website contains a customizable slide presentation on credentialing and privileging basics that can be used for orienting board members with regard to these issues. The following are areas of the medical staff bylaws that address the governing body:

- **MS.01.01.01:** The governing body must approve and comply with medical staff bylaws. The bylaws, rules and regulations, and policies of the medical staff cannot conflict with the governing body bylaws. Both medical staff and board bylaws may address the same issues (e.g., credentialing and privileging). At times, changes are made in one body's bylaws, but not the other. Review both medical staff and governing body bylaws and compare to make sure no discrepancies exist. The medical staff must have a process to manage any conflicts that may arise between the medical staff and the MEC regarding recommendations to adopt or change rules, regulations, or policies and other issues that may occur. Medical staff members must have a mechanism, as determined by the governing body, for communicating to the governing body regarding a rule, regulation, or policy adopted by the MEC or by the organized medical staff.

- **MS.01.01.03:** This standard prohibits both the medical staff and the hospital board from changing the medical staff bylaws or rules and regulations without the other group's approval. The Joint Commission has provided literature indicating that an issue such as unilateral amendment of bylaws is a sign that there has been a breakdown in the required collaborative relationship of the medical staff and governing body. The surveyor may question medical staff and hospital leaders regarding the amendment process and specifically ask whether either body has unilaterally amended the medical staff bylaws or rules and regulations.

- **MS.04.01.01:** There must be a mechanism that facilitates effective communication between the graduate medical education (GME) committee (GMEC), the medical staff, and the governing body. This communication must include the safety and quality of patient care, treatment, and services provided by the GME participants, as well as the educational and supervisory needs of the participants. If the GME program extends to a local hospital or other organization, the person(s) responsible for oversight of the program must communicate effectively with the medical staff and governing body. This function can be accomplished in a number of ways. A hospital representative can participate in GMEC meetings or routine written reports can be made to the GMEC. When making these reports, any concerns regarding the care provided by those in the GME program should be reported. Likewise, if there are educational needs that need to be met—for instance, if residents are rotating through a service and there is an obvious need for additional education—bring up this issue. These concerns don't have to wait for a meeting or a formal report. Any time there is a concern, the responsible hospital representative should communicate this to the program director. (This standard pertains to hospitals that participate in GME programs when the graduate will be an LIP. It does not apply to programs that train physician assistants or other types of advanced practice professionals who require direct supervision of an LIP.)

- **MS.05.01.03:** This standard requires the medical staff to participate in organization-wide PI activities. The findings, conclusions, recommendations, and actions to improve performance must be communicated to appropriate staff members and the governing body. Documentation of this review should be included in governing body meeting minutes.

- **MS.06.01.03:** The governing body approves the credentialing process. This is typically done with the board's approval of the medical staff bylaws. If changes are made in the medical staff's process, they should be reflected in the bylaws and provided to the governing body for approval.

- **MS.06.01.05 and MS.06.01.07:** The hospital establishes the criteria used to determine a practitioner's ability to provide patient care, treatment, and services within the scope of the requested privileges and criteria used in the decision to grant, limit, or deny a requested privilege. These criteria must be based on the medical staff's recommendations and approved by the governing body. Criteria are typically included in the medical staff bylaws, but may also be contained in board bylaws. Check for consistency. Final authority for granting, renewing, or denying privileges rests with the governing body or a committee to which the governing body has delegated this function.

- **MS.06.01.11:** An expedited process for appointment/reappointment and privileges can be used by the organization. Although this is addressed in the MS standards, the expedited approval process is actually a function of the governing body. The Joint Commission allows expedited credentialing by enabling the governing body to delegate appointment and privileging decisions to a committee consisting of at least two voting governing body members. Some refer to this process as "fast-track" credentialing. The medical staff must develop specific criteria if it chooses to allow expedited credentialing. As you are evaluating your credentialing processes, if you find there are delays in the board approval process, you may want to consider an expedited credentialing process. See Figure 2.1 for a sample expedited credentialing policy and procedure.

- **MS.07.01.01:** Medical staff membership is granted by the governing body on recommendation of the medical staff. Note that there are separate standards regarding board approvals—one for membership and one for privileges. Each of these should be reported separately in board minutes with language such as, "Members considered the recommendations from the medical staff regarding new applicants and it moved, seconded, and carried to approve medical staff membership and clinical privileges as requested." Some organizations also like to use a form such as the "Recommendation and Approval Form for Medical Staff Appointment and Clinical Privileges" (Figure 2.2), which is contained on this book's downloadable resource page.

- **MS.09.01.01:** Pursuant to its bylaws, the medical staff evaluates and acts on reported concerns regarding the clinical practice or competence of a privileged practitioner. The hospital clearly defines the process used for collecting, investigating, and addressing clinical practice concerns regarding privileged practitioners. This process is based on recommendations by the medical staff and approval of the governing body. This EP contains a (D) icon, meaning the surveyor will be looking for documentation of the required process to determine compliance. Although this standard is scored as a MS standard, The Joint Commission assigns responsibility for it to the hospital as a whole. The medical staff can approve and provide input and feedback into the hospital's policy.

<table>
<tr><td>**2.1**</td><td>**Sample Medical Staff Expedited Credentialing Policy and Procedure**</td></tr>
</table>

Purpose:

This policy and procedure is made for rendering appointment, reappointment, and privileging decisions through an expedited credentialing process without compromising the quality of the review. "Expedited credentialing" provides an expedited review and approval process if specific, predefined criteria are met.

Expedited credentialing is neither a right nor a privilege. Candidates who do not meet the criteria for expedited credentialing will be processed through the usual credentialing process as specified in the medical staff bylaws.

Procedure:

The department chair and medical staff coordinator or their designee(s) will review each application, its associated documentation, and the information acquired during the credentialing and privileging process to determine eligibility.

To be eligible for expedited approval, the following criteria must be met:

- The application is complete and accurate with all requested information returned. (A complete application is one in which the application and all primary source verification and information required by the medical staff bylaws are complete.)
- There are no discrepancies in information received and no negative or questionable information is received.
- Medical staff/work history is unremarkable (i.e., no frequent moves or unexplained or alarming gaps).
- The applicant's request for clinical privileges is consistent with the medical staff's designation for the applicant's specialty and his or her experience, training, and current competency; in addition, all applicable privileging criteria are met.
- The applicant possesses a current, valid state license; professional liability insurance in limits specified by the medical staff; and federal/state narcotics certificate(s), if applicable.
- The applicant has indicated that he or she can safely and competently exercise the clinical privileges requested, with or without a reasonable accommodation.
- The applicant's history shows an ability to relate to others in a harmonious, collegial manner.

2.1	Sample Medical Staff Expedited Credentialing Policy and Procedure *(cont.)*

- At the time of renewal of privileges, documentation of activity in the hospital and/or verification from outside healthcare entities/peers sufficiently verifies current competence.
- At the time of renewal of privileges, the results of peer review activities and the quality improvement functions of the medical staff reveal no areas of concern.

Each of the following criteria will be thoroughly evaluated on a case-by-case basis and may lead to ineligibility for expedited credentialing:

- The applicant's medical staff appointment, staff status, and/or clinical privileges have never been involuntarily resigned, denied, revoked, suspended, restricted, reduced, surrendered, or not renewed at any other healthcare facility.
- The applicant has never withdrawn an application for appointment, reappointment, or clinical privileges or resigned from the medical staff before a decision was made by another healthcare facility's governing board or to avoid denial or termination of such.
- No licenses; DEA or other controlled-substance authorizations; membership in local, state, or national professional societies; or board certification have ever been suspended, modified, terminated, or voluntarily or involuntarily surrendered.
- The applicant has not been named as a defendant in a criminal action or been convicted of a crime.
- There are no significant adverse findings reported by the National Practitioner Data Bank, Healthcare Practitioner Data Bank, Federation of State Medical Boards, the AMA/American Osteopathic Association, or any other practitioner database.
- There are no past or pending malpractice actions, including claims, lawsuits, arbitrations, settlements, awards, or judgments, that show an unusual pattern of, or an excessive number of, professional liability actions resulting in a final judgment against the applicant.
- There are no proposed or actual exclusions and/or any pending investigations of the applicant from any healthcare program funded in whole or in part by the federal government, including Medicare or Medicaid.

	Sample Medical Staff Expedited Credentialing
2.1	Policy and Procedure *(cont.)*

Processing of applications:

The following should take place as part of the processing of applications:

1. The medical staff office receives and processes the application according to organization and medical staff policy.

If, at any point in the application processing process, any reviewer feels that the application does not meet criteria for expedited credentialing, the file will be processed and transmitted through the full review process as outlined in the medical staff bylaws.

2. The appropriate department chair or designee reviews the completed and verified application and forwards a report with findings and a recommendation to the medical executive committee (MEC).

3. The MEC reviews the application at its next scheduled meeting and forwards its recommendation to the governing body's credentials committee.

4. The governing body's credentials committee reviews and evaluates the qualifications and competence of the practitioner applying for appointment, reappointment, or renewal or modification of clinical privileges and renders its decision. A positive decision results in the appointment or privileges requested. The date of the committee's decision is the approval date, or the committee may assign an "effective" approval date.

If the decision is adverse to an applicant, the matter will be referred back to the MEC for further evaluation. The governing body's credentials committee will report its recommendation to the full board.

2.2	Recommendation and Approval Form for Medical Staff Appointment and Clinical Privileges

Practitioner Name: _____

Staff Status: _____   Department: _____   Specialty: _____

Departmental Recommendation

Based on the evaluation of the education, training, current competence, health status, skill, character, and judgment of the applicant, the following recommendations are made:

❑ Privileges be granted/renewed

❑ Medical staff membership be granted/renewed

❑ Additional privileges requested be granted

❑ Privileges be modified as follows: _____

_____

❑ Privileges not be granted/renewed

❑ Medical staff membership not be granted/renewed (comment below)

❑ Additional privileges requested be denied (comment below)

Comments: _____

_____   _____
Department Chair   Date

Credentials Committee Recommendation

Based on the evaluation of the education, training, current competence, health status, skill, character, and judgment of the applicant and on the evaluations and recommendations of the department chair, the following recommendations are made:

❑ Concur with recommendation(s) of the department chair and forward these recommendations to the medical executive committee

2.2 Recommendation and Approval Form for Medical Staff Appointment and Clinical Privileges *(cont.)*

❑ Do not concur with the recommendations of the department chair and instead make the following recommendations:

_____

_____

_____   _____
Credentials Committee Representative   Date

Medical Staff Executive Committee Recommendation

Based on the evaluation of the education, training, current competence, health status, skill, character, and judgment of the applicant and on the evaluations and recommendations of the department chair and credentials committee, the following recommendations are made:

❑ Concur with recommendation(s) of the department chairman and credentials committee and forward these recommendations to the governing body for consideration

❑ Do not agree with the recommendations of the department chair and credentials committee and instead make the following recommendations:

_____

_____

_____   _____
Medical Staff Executive Committee Representative   Date

Governing Body Approvals/Action Taken

Based on the evaluation of the education, training, current competence, health status, skill, character, and judgment data and information, and on the recommendations of the medical staff, the following action is taken:

❑ Concur with and approve the recommendation(s) of the medical staff.

❑ Do not concur with the recommendations of the medical staff. Action taken is documented in board minutes of _____.

                            (date)

_____   _____
Board of Trustees Representative   Date

- **MS.10.01.01:** There must be mechanisms for a fair hearing and appeals process to address adverse decisions regarding reappointment, denial, reduction, suspension, or revocation of privileges that may relate to quality of care, treatment, and services issues. The standard does not state that all adverse decisions should trigger the fair hearing process—only those that relate to quality of care, treatment, and services issues. Automatic suspensions for issues such as failing to complete medical records and not completing applications on time need not trigger a hearing or appeal. The mechanisms must allow the affected individual a fair opportunity for defense of the alleged wrongs to an unbiased hearing body of the medical staff. There also must be a mechanism by which to appeal the decision of the hearing body to the governing body. Check governing body bylaws for documentation of this appeal mechanism.

Medical staff

Medical staff members are typically not aware of their responsibilities under Joint Commission standards. Although oversight of the medical staff is the responsibility of medical staff leaders, it is typically up to the hospital staff to make sure they are aware of the standards and that they are complying with them. In the next chapter, we will break down the individual standards and provide some ideas and tools to help with compliance.

Some organizational requirements regarding the medical staff are contained in the Leadership chapter of the standards. As such, you may wish to read the companion book on the Leadership chapter for more insight into these standards.

PART 3

Medical Staff Standards: Implementation

Now that we know the key players, it's time to break down the standards and review some mechanisms for implementing the requirements.

What Is the Impact on Patient Care of the Medical Staff Standards?

The medical staff (MS) standards have a significant impact on patient care. This section covers credentialing, privileging, and oversight of medical staff and others providing patient care, treatment, and services. Licensed independent practitioners (LIP) must apply for medical staff appointment and clinical privileges, and the care they provide must be continually monitored. The standards cover the processes that must be followed when performing these essential functions. The standards are designed to result in patient care being provided by competent and qualified practitioners, lessening the chance of poor or adverse patient outcomes.

How Are Processes Successfully Maintained?

The medical staff must be well-organized to participate actively in important organizational functions. To accomplish this goal, the medical staff develops and adopts bylaws, rules, regulations, and other policies and defines its organizational structure in a way that allows it to accomplish its responsibilities. Medical staffs have either elected or appointed officers. They typically are separated into departments that reflect physician specialties or subspecialties. Each of these departments, in turn, will have elected or appointed officers conduct its meetings. In most cases, physician department directors assume administrative responsibilities in addition to their patient care responsibilities. They may or may not get paid for this additional work.

Committees that make recommendations to the medical staff executive committee carry out many of the medical staff's required functions. They perform many functions required by The Joint Commission and other regulatory bodies on behalf of the medical staff. They also evaluate and make recommendations regarding clinical processes and organizational functions. Medical staff meetings are a great tool for brainstorming on important issues.

Credentialing, privileging, and oversight processes must be consistently applied. Bylaws, rules, regulations, policies, and procedures must be reviewed for compliance with standards and to make sure they are being followed and are current and comprehensive. Bylaws, rules and regulations of the hospital governing body, and those of the medical staff should not conflict.

Medical services professionals (MSP) support the duties of medical staff leaders by helping them develop criteria for appointment, privileges, and reappointment. They also perform the credentialing function, manage medical staff meetings, orient medical staff leaders and applicants, maintain and update bylaws, and serve as a resource to the medical staff and its leaders.

Medical staff offices (MSO) must be adequately staffed with properly educated and trained personnel to effectively and efficiently meet the needs of the organized medical staff. The issue of staffing the MSO is significant since credentialing and privileging are essential functions that carry a considerable amount of risk to both patient safety and the hospital if not performed to the generally recognized standard. This is evidenced by an increased number of negligent credentialing lawsuits as well as Centers for Medicare & Medicaid Services' (CMS) Interpretive Guidelines that reflect an increased scrutiny of hospital credentialing and privileging processes. As such, the importance of the job of those performing medical staff support functions cannot be overstated MSPs require adequate computer hardware/software and office equipment as well. Organization support for continuing education is essential.

What Activities/Requirements/Policies/Procedures Are Affected, and What Is Done to Make Sure This Happens Successfully?

There are a number of required policies and procedures referenced in the MS standards. The next section will break down the standards and provide some sample policies, procedures, and tools that can be utilized to meet the standards.

The chart that follows is included on the tools website and can be used for documenting areas in need of improvement.

3.1	Chart for Documenting Recommendations

Standard & EP number	Type of issue (check all that apply)			Related MS document/ process	Involved individuals	Suggestions for resolving issue	Date resolved
	Noncompliance with standard due to written policy/procedure deficiency	Noncompliance due to inadequately applying current policy	Opportunity for improvement				

Breakdown of the Medical Staff Standards

Each of the medical staff standards is included in this summary, but they may not appear in numerical order. Like standards are grouped together for the benefit of easy reading.

In addition, some standards apply only to hospitals that use Joint Commission accreditation for deemed status purposes. This means they apply to hospitals that use Joint Commission accreditation in lieu of the routine state surveys for Medicare and Medicaid participation.

MS.01.01.01: Organized medical staff structure, accountability, and bylaws (effective March 2011)

MS.01.01.01 requires the medical staff bylaws to speak to self-governance and the medical staff's accountability to the governing body. It spells out specific items that must appear in

the medical staff bylaws and what can be included in other documents, such as policies, procedures, rules, and regulations. Joint Commission surveyors will expect medical staff leaders to know the process for approval and amendment of bylaws and other medical staff documents.

The organized medical staff develops, adopts, and amends bylaws. The process for adoption and amendment cannot be delegated. Proposed changes in bylaws must be submitted to the governing body for action and do not become effective until approved.

You can create a helpful tool by including a summary sheet in the bylaws, such as the one in Figure 3.2, with all changes made in medical staff manuals. It will provide a quick reference to all changes made by your facility.

Medical staff bylaws, rules and regulations, and policies can be proposed directly to the governing body. If the medical staff chooses to do this, it should first convey the proposed change to the medical executive committee (MEC).

3.2	Sample Change Implementation Chart	

Date of board approval	Manual	Article/section modified
7/22/10	Bylaws	Article II, Section A.2
9/24/10	Bylaws	Article V, Section G.5
10/27/10	Bylaws	Article X, Section 7
10/27/10	Rules and regulations	Part 10, Section 5.L
1/22/11	Rules and regulations	Part 6, Section 4
2/24/11	Bylaws	Article V, Section 5.B.3

The medical staff may choose to delegate authority to make proposals for changes in rules, regulations, or policies to the MEC. When the MEC recommends a change or amendment to rules, regulations, policies, or procedures, the proposed changes should be communicated to the medical staff. (This only applies if the organized medical staff has delegated this authority to the MEC and the governing body has approved the delegation.)

The medical staff must have a process to manage any conflicts that may arise between the medical staff and the MEC regarding recommendations to adopt or change rules, regulations, or policies and other issues that may occur. (See the sample conflict management process language in Figure 3.3.)

Using a mechanism determined by the governing body, medical staff members may communicate to the governing body regarding a rule, regulation, or policy adopted by the MEC or by the organized medical staff. The leadership standards also require the medical staff and governing board to develop a conflict resolution process.

There may be an incidence in which a critical change to rules and regulations may be necessary in order to comply with law or regulation. In these cases, there can be a process for the MEC to provisionally adopt and the board to provisionally approve these amendments without notifying the medical staff. This authority must be delegated by the voting members of the organized medical staff. If this urgent amendment is required, the MEC must immediately notify the medical staff of the change, and the medical staff must be given the opportunity for retrospective review and comment. If the medical staff and MEC are in agreement, the amendment stands, but if there is a disagreement, the conflict resolution process is implemented.

3.3	Sample Conflict Management Process Language

If a conflict arises between the Medical Executive Committee and the Medical Staff regarding the adoption, amendment, or deletion of medical staff bylaws, recommendations to adopt or change rules, regulations, or policies, or any other conflicting issues, medical staff leaders, the medical executive committee, hospital senior leadership, and the governing body should work as a team to manage the conflict. The process may include the use of external resources or a hospital employee trained in conflict management to help facilitate the process. If a resolution cannot be reached through this information mechanism, the issue will be referred to a Joint Conference Committee of the Board and Medical Staff.

Joint Conference Committee

A. Composition: The Joint Conference Committee shall consist of three members of the Executive Committee of the Board and three members of the Medical Staff Executive Committee. The Chair of the Board shall serve as the chairman. The Medical Director and Hospital CEO shall serve as ex officio members of the committee without vote.

B. Duties: The Joint Conference Committee's duties shall include:

   a. To act as a forum for the discussion of medico-administrative matters;

   b. To review and consider issues that may arise in the planning and operation of the Hospital that may affect the relationship among the Board, the Medical Staff, and the Hospital Senior Leadership;

   c. To manage any areas of conflict between the Board, the Medical Staff, and the Hospital Senior Leadership that may arise, including the adoption, amendment, or deletion of medical staff bylaws, and recommendations to adopt or change rules, regulations, or policies.

C. Meeting frequency: The Joint Conference Committee shall meet as necessary to accomplish its duties.

The medical staff must comply with and enforce, and the governing body must uphold, the bylaws, policies, and procedures. The medical staff may do this by recommending to the governing body that specific action is taken, and in some cases, the medical staff may have authority to take action itself.

Medical staff bylaws, rules and regulations, and policies must not conflict with the governing body bylaws. Coordination is necessary between the medical staff and the governing body in this area. Both entities' documents typically spell out changes in medical staff structure and credentialing and privileging processes. Both entities should have ready access to these documents. When making a change to either, evaluate both documents to make sure there are no conflicts. Figure 3.4 contains a sample form for creating a crosswalk between medical staff and governing body bylaws.

Bylaws must conform to state and federal regulations. Because each state has its own licensing regulations, these regulations should be reviewed to make sure all required elements are

3.4	Crosswalk Medical Staff and Governing Bylaws, Rules, Regulations, Policies, and Procedures [Hospital Name]	
MEDICAL STAFF DOCUMENT	**ISSUE ADDRESSED**	**BOARD DOCUMENT**
Article V, Section 1.3	Medical staff representation on governing body	Article II, Section 2.3

included. For example, state regulations may require bylaws to include specific time frames (e.g., 60 days) for completing the credentialing process. Joint Commission surveyors will expect this to be specified in the bylaws.

The following elements are required to be addressed in medical staff bylaws. In some cases, there may be some related details or fine points that, according to the medical staff's preference, may be contained in the medical staff bylaws, or may be in rules, regulations, or policies. Although authority for adoption of associated details contained in bylaws can't be delegated, the medical can delegate the adoption of changes to details contained in rules, regulations, or policies. At a minimum, basic steps in required processes must be delineated in bylaws.

For example, the process for approving grants of clinical privileges, to be spelled out in the bylaws, might include department chair review and recommendation, MEC review and recommendation, and governing body approval. The procedure the hospital uses to collect all information necessary to document competency for privilege requests may be contained in rules and regulations or a policy and procedure. Review your bylaws to make sure all required elements are included, paying particular attention to ensuring that basic steps for all required processes are included in the bylaws. A tool entitled "Chart for Review of Bylaws for Compliance With The Joint Commission Standards Required Documentation" is provided on the Tools website for evaluation of your bylaws.

- Medical staff structure. A typical structure includes the officers, departments, committees, etc., as well as which providers are eligible for medical staff membership.

- Qualifications to be met in order to be appointed to the medical staff. Typical criteria include such things as specified education, training, licensure, professional liability coverage, etc.

- The duties and privileges for each medical staff category of the medical staff (e.g., active, courtesy). This is a requirement of CMS' *Conditions of Participation*. The Joint Commission interprets this to mean "the duties and prerogatives of each category," not clinical privileges that are typically delineated on a privilege form.

- Requirements for completing and documenting histories and physicals (H&P). This is a requirement of CMS' *Conditions of Participation*. H&Ps must be completed and documented by a physician, an oral maxillofacial surgeon, or other qualified licensed individual. State law and hospital policy must be followed. Check to make sure that bylaws include a requirement that the patient receives the H&P no more than 30 days prior to, or within 24 hours after registration or inpatient admission, and prior to surgery or a procedure requiring anesthesia. Also check to make sure that for an H&P completed within 30 days prior to registration or inpatient admission, an update documenting any changes in the patient's condition is required to be completed within 24 hours after registration or inpatient admission and prior to surgery or a procedure requiring anesthesia.

- Description of medical staff members eligible to vote.

- Medical staff officer positions.

- Function, size, and composition of the MEC. If authority is delegated to the MEC to act on behalf of the medical staff, such authority is documented as is the mechanism for delegation or removal of this authority.

- Documentation that the MEC includes physicians and may include others if established by the medical staff.

- Documentation that the MEC has authority to act on behalf of the medical staff between meetings. This happens within the defined responsibilities of the MEC.

- Indications for:

  - Automatic suspension and summary suspension of medical staff membertship or clinical privileges.

  - Recommending termination or suspension of medical staff membership and/or termination, suspension, or reduction of clinical privileges.

  - Note: An automatic suspension is an administrative action that occurs when a physician fails to comply with a medical staff rule (e.g., clinical privileges suspension due to noncompliance with medical records completion requirements). A summary suspension is imposed pursuant to bylaws requirements for such an action. For example, if a physician appears to be intoxicated while making patient rounds, he or she could be summarily suspended for patient safety reasons while the incident is under investigation.

- Processes for:

  - Credentialing/recredentialing and privileging/reprivileging LIPs and other practitioners

  - Medical staff appointment and reappointment

  - Selecting, electing, and removing MEC members

- Adopting and amending the medical staff bylaws, rules and regulations, and policies

- Fair hearing and appeal of an adverse recommendation including how hearings and appeals are scheduled and conducted and the composition of the hearing committee

- Selection, election, and removal of medical staff officers

- Automatic and summary suspension of medical staff membership or clinical privileges

- Recommending termination or suspension of medical staff membership and/or termination, suspension, or reduction of clinical privileges

- If the medical staff is departmentalized, the qualifications, roles, and responsibilities of the department chair must be included. Standards include a comprehensive list of the roles and responsibilities of the department chair. (See Part 2 for the roles and responsibilities of the department chair.) The chair must be certified by an appropriate specialty board or the comparable competence affirmatively established through the credentialing process. That is, if your medical staff wants to allow nonboard certified members to function as department chairs, you must define competency criteria. For instance, the following could serve as sample language:

  - "Department chairs must be members in good standing with no disciplinary action, have served as an officer of the department for at least two years, and be board certified or possess comparable competence to an individual with board certification. Comparable competence is defined as at least five years of active staff membership with major privileges with evaluation under the medical staff's quality assessment process showing quality patient care."

MS.01.01.03: Bylaws amendments

MS.01.01.03 prohibits both the medical staff and the hospital board from changing the medical staff bylaws or rules and regulations without the other group's approval. The Joint Commission's published materials indicate that an issue such as unilateral amendment of bylaws is a sign that there has been a breakdown in the required collaborative relationship of the medical staff and governing body. The surveyor may question medical staff and hospital leaders regarding the amendment process and specifically ask whether either body has unilaterally amended the medical staff bylaws or rules and regulations.

MS.02.01.01: Medical executive committee

MS.02.01.01 requires that an MEC be formed. The individual EPs describe the functions, composition, and responsibilities of the MEC and what needs to be documented in medical staff bylaws. Your hospital's medical staff is free to define the structure. It may be composed of elected or appointed department directors or it may be a body of elected members. In a hospital with a small medical staff, the medical staff as a whole may serve as the executive committee. In this case, the medical staff is known as a "committee of the whole."

The structure and function of the MEC must conform to what is documented in the medical staff bylaws. In scoring this standard, the surveyor may compare a listing of the actual committee members with the requirements in the bylaws to determine whether they are consistent. The hospital's CEO or designee attends each MEC meeting. This occurs on an ex officio basis, with or without a vote. The majority of voting members of the MEC must be fully licensed physicians who are practicing actively in the hospital. Regardless of specialty or discipline, all members of the organized medical staff must be eligible for MEC membership. This means that if your medical staff grants membership to advanced practice nurses or other

LIPs, then these categories of practitioners should be eligible for MEC membership. In intervals between medical staff meetings, the MEC acts on behalf of the medical staff.

The MEC must have a mechanism by which to recommend terminations of medical staff membership. When there is a question about the ability to perform the privileges granted for a practitioner privileged through the medical staff process, the MEC must request an evaluation of that practitioner.

The MEC has the authority to make recommendations and must make recommendations to the governing body regarding the structure of the medical staff.

The MEC's authority to make recommendations to the governing body regarding medical staff membership must be defined in the bylaws, and this must be done in practice.

The MEC must make recommendations to the governing body regarding delineation of privileges for individual practitioners as well as the process used for delineation of privileges for all practitioners who are privileged through the medical staff process. This includes practitioners such as advanced practice nurses and physician assistants who are granted privileges without being granted medical staff appointment.

As defined in the bylaws, the MEC must make recommendations to the governing body regarding the MEC's authority to review and act on the reports of medical staff committees, departments, and other groups or committees.

MS.03.01.01: Oversight of practitioners

The medical staff must oversee the quality of patient care, treatment, and services provided by all practitioners who are privileged through the medical staff process. Medical staff oversight functions must be assigned to LIPs who are medical staff members. In other words, if the medical staff includes practitioners other than LIPs, these non-LIPs are not assigned any oversight activities.

The medical staff defines the scope of privileges for all practitioners, and practitioners must practice only within the scope of their privileges. The organization must have a mechanism for ensuring that practitioners are only performing procedures for which they have privileges.

The medical staff uses documented processes to provide leadership in activities that relate to patient safety. Patient safety is a major focus of The Joint Commission. Surveyors will be looking for specific examples of how the medical staff participates in this function.

The medical staff must participate in the oversight of the analysis and improvement of patient satisfaction processes. Compliance with this standard can be documented by presenting summaries of the results of patient surveys at the MEC meetings.

The medical staff must specify the minimum content for H&P examinations and must monitor the quality of H&P exams. Even though the medical staff may set minimum guidelines for what needs to be included, there will still be considerable variability in the format and content of the H&P, depending on the clinical judgment of the practitioner and the care that is being provided. For example, if a patient is having outpatient surgery to remove surgical screws inserted during a previous orthopedic repair, the relevant and pertinent H&P exam might include current patient condition and vital signs, the history of the trauma or activity that resulted in the surgical repair and subsequent removal of screws, any cardiac or respiratory history, and current medications. In addition to the information the medical staff requires in the H&P, the medical staff should evaluate whether the H&P is pertinent, relevant, and includes sufficient information to provide care and services and meet the needs of that specific patient.

H&Ps are only performed by practitioners who have been granted privileges by the hospital to do so. The medical staff may allow individuals other than LIPs to perform part or all of a patient's H&P. However, this work must be performed under supervision of, or through delegation by, a physician who is responsible for the H&P. It is only allowed if permitted by state law and medical staff policy. Note that this standard refers to privileges granted by the hospital, not by the medical staff. Evaluate this closely, especially if the hospital allows physician assistants and advanced practice nurses who are credentialed and privileged through the alternative process specified in the Human Resources standards to perform these exams. Make sure everyone who is performing H&Ps has the privileges required to do so. Some states specify who can perform these exams. The medical staff must define when an H&P must be validated and countersigned by a responsible, privileged LIP. For outpatient services, the medical staff defines the scope of the H&P. Many hospitals use a short form for H&Ps for outpatient surgery under local anesthesia that includes relevant history and pertinent physical findings. This should be documented.

For hospitals that use Joint Commission accreditation for deemed status purposes, the following standards apply:

- If the hospital provides emergency services but these services are not provided at off-campus locations, there must be documented medical staff policies and procedures for appraising emergencies, providing initial treatment for patients, and facilitating appropriate referral of patients seen at the off-campus locations. If emergency services are not provided at the hospital, the medical staff should develop policies and procedures for appraising emergencies, providing initial treatment for patients, and facilitating referral of patients as appropriate.

- The qualifications of the radiology staff members who utilize equipment and administer procedures and the qualifications, training, functions, and responsibilities of the nuclear medicine staff, as specified by the director of nuclear services, must be approved by the medical staff. These approvals can be accomplished by the medical staff's review and approval of the job descriptions and qualifications. This responsibility can be delegated to the MEC, but authority for this delegation should be included in medical staff bylaws.

MS.03.01.03: Management and oversight of patient care

Patients may be seen by many care providers, depending on the reason for admission. For care to occur in a well-run, safe manner, there must be coordination and communication among all who are providing patient care, treatment, or services. In addition to the hospital's programs, there must be coordination between the practitioner and a hospital to which the patient may be transferred, managed care organizations for issues of utilization review, and the patient and family.

Each patient's care, treatment, and services must be managed and coordinated by LIPs with appropriate privileges. Although specific services and treatments may be delegated to nonphysician LIPs, a doctor of medicine or osteopathy must manage and coordinate the patient's general medical condition. For hospitals that use Joint Commission accreditation for deemed status purposes, an MD or DO must manage and coordinate psychiatric problems not specifically within the scope of practice of an oral surgeon, dentist, podiatrist, optometrist, chiropractor, or clinical psychologist.

The medical staff specifies when consultation and management by a physician or other LIP is required, and consultation is to be obtained in all circumstances required by the medical staff. This can be documented in medical staff bylaws, rules, regulations, and policies. In addition, clinical practice guidelines and privilege forms may specify when consultation is necessary. This can also apply to a specific setting, such as the ICU. Some hospitals use a form, such as the one in Figure 3.5. All practitioners involved with a patient's care, treatment, and services coordinate that care, treatment, and services.

All LIPs must be educated by the hospital in assessing and managing pain. Some ways of doing this include:

- Using a continuous-loop PowerPoint® presentation with your hospital's current pain procedures and running it prior to medical staff meetings or in the doctors' lounge

- Presentation by pain management providers at medical staff meetings

- Include in physician orientation

- Publish information in newsletter or other form of written communication

For hospitals that use Joint Commission accreditation for deemed status purposes, there must be an MD or DO either on call or on duty at all times.

3.5	Sample Clinical Consultation Form

Request for clinical consultation

Date of request: _____

Date of initial patient visit by clinical consultant: _____

Attending (requesting) physician: _____

Clinical consultant: _____

The following information is to be completed by the requesting physician.

Reason(s) for requesting clinical consultation:

_____ Diagnosis obscure

_____ Patient not responding to treatment as expected

_____ Patient or family requests clinical consultation or a second opinion

_____ Other _____

_____

_____

Please:

_____ Evaluate the patient and discuss findings and suggestions with me

_____ Evaluate the patient, discuss findings and suggestions with me, and follow up with me

_____ Assume care of the patient

_____

Requesting physician's signature

Note: Place this form in the patient's medical record.

MS.04.01.01: Graduate medical education programs

This standard pertains to hospitals that participate in GME programs when the graduate will be an LIP. It does not apply to programs that train physician assistants or other types of advanced practice professionals who require direct supervision of an LIP. If your hospital does not participate in these programs, this standard does not apply to your hospital and you can skip this section.

The medical staff must define the process used for supervising each participant of the GME program in carrying out patient care responsibilities. This supervision is the responsibility of an LIP who has appropriate clinical privileges. This standard contains the "D" icon, which requires documentation to determine compliance.

The medical staff and hospital staff must be provided with written descriptions of the roles, responsibilities, and patient care activities of GME participants and the mechanisms by which the GME participant's program director and supervisors make decisions regarding the participant's increased involvement and independence in specific patient care activities. Typically, attending staff determines the level of responsibility accorded to each resident based on direct observation and knowledge of each resident's skills and abilities. This level may vary with the clinical circumstances.

The medical staff defines which GME participants can write patient care orders, and under what circumstances, in rules, regulations, and policies. This requirement must not prohibit LIPs from writing orders. (For instance, in a fellowship program, the participants may be LIPs already.) The medical staff also must define what entries a supervising LIP must countersign.

There must be a mechanism for communicating between the GME committee, the medical staff, and the governing body. This is true regardless of whether the training occurs at the hospital that sponsors the GME program or at a local or community hospital that participates in the program. Communication must include the safety and quality of patient care, treatment, and services provided by the GME participants, as well as the educational and supervisory needs of the participants. Any time there is a concern, the responsible hospital representative should communicate this to the program director. If the residency review committee issues a citation, the medical staff must be able to show that it is in compliance with the citation.

MS.05.01.01: Medical staff performance improvement

To improve the quality of care, treatment, and services and to increase patient safety, the medical staff must take a leadership role in hospital performance improvement (PI) activities. Information relevant to key hospital processes must be incorporated into the PI activities. During this process, confidentiality and privilege of information must be maintained.

The medical staff develops and adopts a PI plan to provide written guidelines used to monitor and continually improve the processes performed by LIPs and others privileged through the medical staff process. Medical staff leaders should have intimate knowledge of this PI plan and be ready to discuss it with surveyors.

The medical staff must be actively involved in measuring, assessing, and improving the following critical organizational processes (active involvement can include review of charts, analyzing data, and attending PI meetings):

- Medical assessments (H&Ps) and treatments ordered or provided.

- How the medical staff will use any information concerning adverse privileging decisions for those privileged through the medical staff process. The privileging function of the medical staff may identify areas in which improvement is needed. For instance, focused evaluation of patient outcomes for a specific procedure may determine that practitioners with a specialized level of training perform the procedure more efficiently and with better patient outcomes. For this reason, the medical staff may decide to limit performance of this procedure to those with the specialized training. This decision would mean that practitioners who do not have the specialized training would have their privileges reduced.

- Appropriate use of medications. This function is often accomplished through a pharmacy and therapeutics committee. Be ready to show the minutes of these meetings to the surveyor, as well as any recommendations that came from this evaluation and the follow-up to these recommendations.

- Ordering and administration of blood and blood components. The PI standards require the hospital to gather and evaluate high-risk procedures, including the administration of blood and blood components. Blood components include red blood cells, platelets, plasma, cryoprecipitate, and granulocytes. The medical staff develops appropriateness criteria, which include the indications for administration of each product used in the hospital setting and review of those cases that do not meet the indications.

- Operative and other procedures. This includes indications for procedures, complications, and pathological review of tissue removed for both procedures performed in the operating room and diagnostic procedures performed in areas such as vascular and endoscopy suites and cardiac catheterization laboratories.

- Appropriateness of clinical practice patterns. As this standard implies, the medical staff must analyze clinical practice patterns for LIPs and other providers privileged through the medical staff function.

- Any significant deviations from established patterns of clinical practice.

- How developed criteria for autopsies are used. The medical staff should define when an autopsy is required. If the hospital uses Joint Commission accreditation for deeming purposes, it must attempt to obtain autopsies in cases in which there is an unusual death and in cases of medical, legal, and educational interest. It must also inform the attending physician (or clinical psychologist) if the hospital plans to perform an autopsy on his or her patient.

- Data regarding sentinel events are included as part of the PI process, A sentinel event is defined by The Joint Commission as an unexpected occurrence involving death or serious physical/psychological injury, or the risk of such an injury. A serious injury is defined as one that includes the loss of a limb or function. When evaluating the phrase "or the risk thereof," The Joint Commission includes any process variation that could result in a significant chance of a serious adverse outcome. The Joint Commission also references a "near miss." This term describes a process variation that did not negatively affect an outcome but that, if it were to recur, would carry a significant chance of a serious adverse outcome. A near miss is considered a sentinel event, but it is not subject to review under The Joint Commission's sentinel event policy.

- Patient safety data are included as part of the PI process. This standard is also reflected in the leadership standards, which require implementation of an organizationwide integrated patient safety program.

MS.05.01.03: Medical staff participation in organizational performance improvement

This standard requires the medical staff to participate in organizationwide PI activities. Hospitals develop and adopt PI programs that establish a formal, organizationwide system to monitor and continuously improve patient outcomes and client services.

The medical staff must be involved in the overall PI activities for the organization, not just those related to the medical staff, including:

- Educating patients and their families. The medical staff can document involvement by developing patient educational brochures and videos and taking part in patient informational lectures.

- Coordinating the care, treatment, and services provided to each patient with the other practitioners and hospital personnel who are caring for the patient.

- Completion of medical records that are accurate, timely, and legible. This standard is also reflected and scored in the Record of Care chapter of the standards.

- When the assessment process reveals issues that are relevant to an individual's performance, the medical staff must determine how this information is used in the ongoing evaluation of a practitioner's competence. The PI plan should document how this information is integrated into the medical staff's evaluation process for LIPs. Surveyors will look for instances in which the PI process identified an issue regarding a specific practitioner and the medical staff's follow-up to that issue. They may ask to see information reviewed during the ongoing and focused professional practice review processes or on reappointment to determine whether this issue was considered. Surveyors also may ask to see documents that detail any corrective action that was taken as a result of an issue identified during PI activities.

The findings, conclusions, recommendations, and actions to improve performance must be communicated to appropriate staff members and the governing body. This can be accomplished by forwarding a summary of the recommendations to the board. Generic information not related to specific practitioners can be included in medical staff newsletters, discussion at medical staff department meetings, postings to the medical staff's website, e-mail communications, mailings to specific practitioners, and postings in the medical staff lounges and physician dictation areas.

MS.06.01.01: Determining organizational resource availability

The organization can only grant privileges when the facility has the necessary resources to support the privilege or will have the resources available in a specified time period. The Joint Commission has long required that privileges be setting-specific, meaning that they reflect what the hospital can support in a specific setting.

There is must be a process whereby the hospital consistently determines whether sufficient space, equipment, staffing, and financial resources are in place or will be available within a specified time frame to support each requested privilege. This requires the medical staff and hospital to develop such a process if it does not already exist. This is best done by following a documented procedure. The form included in Figure 3.6 can be used as a tool for developing privileging criteria for a new procedure.

3.6 Worksheet for Consideration of New Privilege

Name of procedure/privilege: _____

Education required to request privilege (check all that apply):

❏ MD - Medical Doctor

❏ DO - Osteopathic Physician

❏ DDS - Oral and Maxillofacial Surgeon

❏ DMD - Dentist

❏ DPM - Podiatrist

❏ APN - Advanced Practice Nurse (specify specialty) _____

❏ PA - Physician Assistant (specify specialty) _____

❏ DC - Chiropractic

❏ Other (specify) _____

Training required: _____

_____

Experience required: _____

_____

Additional requirements:

❏ CME   ❏ Board Certification

❏ Manufacturer's Training Course/Certificate   ❏ Peer Recommendations

Is monitoring or proctoring required?

❏ No   ❏ Yes

If yes, specify the following:

❏ Number of procedures _____   ❏ Length of time _____

❏ In order to complete proctorship/monitoring requirements, the applicant must perform

_____ (number) procedures within _____ (time frame).

What type of review or follow-up will be conducted?

_____

_____

MS.06.01.03: Credentialing

The Joint Commission defines credentialing as a process involving "the collection, verification, and assessment of information regarding three critical parameters: current licensure; education and relevant training; and experience, ability, and current competence to perform the requested privilege(s)." Verification of credentials ensures that the provider's credentials are real and that he or she has the experience and training to perform the privileges requested. The credentialing and privileging process should be an objective and evidence-based process.

The Joint Commission's credentialing and privileging standards reference the six areas of "general competencies" adopted from the Accreditation Council for Graduate Medical Education and the American Board of Medical Specialties (ABMS) joint initiative. These evaluation areas include:

- Patient care and procedural skills

- Medical knowledge

- Practice-based learning and improvement

- Interpersonal and communication skills

- Professionalism

- Systems-based practice

Although not required to be evaluated by Joint Commission standards, many hospitals have chosen to incorporate evaluation of the six areas of general competencies into their credentialing processes; the sample letters and forms that appear in this book reflect these competencies.

Information specific to the applicant's current licensure status, training, experience, competence, and ability to perform the privileges requested must be gathered by the hospital. Note that the standards assign responsibility for this part of the credentialing process to the hospital. Although this seems to conflict with the requirement in MS.01.01.01, which requires the medical staff bylaws to include a description of the credentialing process, it reflects actual practice. The medical staff's definition of the credentialing process typically includes what information is gathered, the process for evaluating that information, and how recommendations are made to the board. The hospital's procedures for carrying out the steps in the process go into much more detail, including which entities and organizations are queried and how those queries are conducted.

Applicants must be credentialed by the hospital using a defined process outlined in the bylaws, based on medical staff recommendations, and approved by the governing body. Note that the standard calls for the process to be outlined. This would not need to include the specific step-by-step process the hospital would use to verify each individual credential.

Practitioner identity must be verified by viewing either a current picture hospital ID card or a valid picture ID issued by a state or federal agency, such as a driver's license or passport. If credentialing a telemedicine provider, have the contracted agency perform the verification and submit documentation to your hospital that the identity was verified. See Figure 3.7 for a sample policy and procedure for verification of identity. This policy and procedure is also included on the Tools website.

3.7	Sample Policy and Procedure for Verification of Identity

Policy:

It is the policy of [Hospital] to verify the identity of all licensed independent practitioners (LIP) who apply for medical staff appointment and privileges prior to the practitioner providing any patient care, treatment, or services. This is done to verify that these practitioners are the same practitioners identified in the credentialing documents.

Verification of identity can be accomplished by viewing any of the following: military ID, state ID, passport, driver's license.

Procedure:

Verification can be done during any of the following processes:

- Provider orientation
- While obtaining hospital picture ID
- Any time the practitioner presents in person to the medical staff office

After presentation of a valid military ID, state driver's license/ID, or customs passport **that includes a picture,** the person verifying completes the Verification of Identity Documentation Form (Attachment A). The completed form is forwarded to the medical staff office for inclusion in the practitioner's credentials file.

Reference: Joint Commission Hospital Standard MS.06.01.03

Attachment A

Verification of Identity Documentation Form

Practitioner Name: _____

I have reviewed the following identification for the above-named practitioner:

❏ Military ID

❏ Passport

❏ State driver's license or ID _____

[list issuing state]

_____	_____	_____
Signature of person verifying	Date	Printed name of person verifying

The medical staff's credentialing process must include a requirement for verification of relevant training, current competence, and current licensure. Verification must be in writing and must come from the primary source, if possible, or from a credentialing verification organization (CVO). Verify licensure at the time of initial granting, renewal, and revision of privileges, and when the license expires.

A primary source is the original issuing source that can verify the accuracy of a credential. For instance, if you are verifying completion of medical school, contact the school for this verification.

The Joint Commission requires primary source verification (PSV) to be in writing, but it can be accomplished via letter, fax, approved official website, or well-documented telephone call. If verifying by phone, include the name of the organization, person providing the information, the questions you asked, and the responses to them. Date and sign the verification.

Designated equivalent sources are agencies that have been determined to maintain a specific item(s) of credential information that is identical to the information at the primary source. A primary source may designate another organization as its agent in providing information to verify credentials. This other organization is then considered a designated equivalent source. The Joint Commission allows the use of designated equivalent sources from which you can obtain information instead of obtaining it directly from the primary source, including the following:

- AMA Physician Masterfile for physician's U.S. and Puerto Rican medical school graduation and residency completion

- ABMS for physician's board certification

- Educational Commission for Foreign Medical Graduates for physician's graduation from a foreign medical school

- American Osteopathic Association (AOA) Physician Database for predoctoral education accredited by the AOA Bureau of Professional Education, postdoctoral education approved by the AOA Council on Postdoctoral Training, and Osteopathic Specialty Board Certification

- Federation of State Medical Boards (FSMB) for actions taken against a physician's medical license

- The American Academy of Physician Assistants Profile for physician assistant education and National Certification Commission on Certification of Physician Assistants for PA certification

Circumstances may not allow you to request or receive information directly from the primary source. For instance, a healthcare facility may close or the applicant's records may be lost or destroyed. Verification of education or training completed in a foreign country may not be accessible. The Joint Commission allows the use of reliable secondary sources after a documented attempt to contact the primary source is made. Another hospital with documented PSV of the applicant's credentials can serve as this secondary source. Examples of secondary source information include written statements from individuals who were in leadership positions in the closed organization or statements from a successor organization. For instance, if a hospital closes and another hospital in the network takes over its credentials files, that hospital can serve as a secondary source.

The Joint Commission allows the use of information received from a CVO to satisfy its requirements for PSV. The Joint Commission has requirements regarding CVOs that are meant to ensure that the hospital has confidence in the accuracy, timeliness, and completeness of the information provided by the CVO. The hospital should evaluate the agency providing the information initially and periodically thereafter. The Joint Commission standards list the following principles to guide hospitals in evaluating CVOs:

- The CVO makes known to the hospital what data and information it can provide.

- The CVO provides documentation describing how its data collection, information and development, and verification process(es) are performed.

- The hospital is provided with information on database functions, including limitations on information available (e.g., practitioners not included in the database), the time frame in which the agency will respond to requests, and an overview of the CVO's quality control processes relating to data integrity, security, transmission accuracy, and technical specifications.

- The CVO and hospital must agree on the format for transmission of an individual's credentials information from the agency.

- The hospital must be able to tell what information transmitted by the agency is from a primary source and what is not.

- For information that may become out of date, the CVO provides the date on which the information was last updated from the primary source.

- The CVO must certify that information transmitted to the hospital accurately represents the information obtained by the CVO.

- The hospital must be able to tell whether the information transmitted by the CVO from a primary source is all the primary source information in the CVO's possession and, if not, where additional information can be obtained.

- When necessary, the hospital can use the CVO's quality control processes to resolve concerns about transmission errors, inconsistencies, or other data issues.

- The hospital must have a formal arrangement with the CVO for communication of any changes in credentialing information.

If your organization uses a CVO, evaluate each of the areas above and list how each aspect is being met. Be prepared to address each aspect of the list with the surveyor.

One additional EP for this standard requires that for hospitals that use Joint Commission accreditation for deemed status purposes, is when a full-time, part-time, or consulting radiologist supervises ionizing radiology services. This MD or DO must be qualified by education and experience in radiology. This standard reflects a CMS requirement.

MS.06.01.05: Privileging

The Joint Commission defines privileging as the "process whereby a specific scope and content of patient care services [clinical privileges] are authorized for a healthcare practitioner by a healthcare organization, based on evaluation of the individual's credentials and performance."

An objective, evidence-based process must be used to grant or deny privileges and when renewing existing privileges. As required by law and regulation, LIPs providing care must have current licensure, certification, or registration.

The hospital establishes the criteria used to determine a practitioner's ability to provide patient care, treatment, and services within the scope of the requested privileges. These criteria must be based on the medical staff's recommendations and approved by the governing body. The hospital must consistently evaluate each criterion for all practitioners with like privileges.

Evidence of physical ability to perform the requested privileges must be evaluated.

Data from professional practice review from the other organization where the applicant currently has privileges must be evaluated if such data are available. This implies that hospitals need to ask for the data to determine whether they are available. Many hospitals consider this information confidential peer review information and will not wish to provide it, but an attempt should be made to get it anyway. Figure 3.8 includes a sample Facility Privileges and Competency Validation letter and form asking for this information, as well as the organization's evaluation of the provider based on the general competencies discussed previously in this chapter.

Criteria for privileges must specify that, on renewal, the medical staff will evaluate the review of the applicant's performance within the hospital.

The evaluation process needs to include consideration of recommendations made by peers and/or faculty. The letter and form in Figure 3.9, Sample Letter for Verification of Training, can be used for obtaining faculty recommendations.

3.8 — Sample Letter Re: Facility Privileges and Competency Validation

Date

Facility Name
Facility Address

Regarding applicant: John Doe, MD
Specialty: General Surgery

Dear Medical Services Professional:

We have received an application from the above-named provider for medical staff appointment and privileges. A copy of the privileges requested is attached. The applicant noted that s/he currently holds, or has in the past held privileges at your facility. In order to process the application, we require documentation of experience, ability, and current competence in the six areas of "general competencies" adopted from the Accreditation Council for Graduate Medical Education and the American Board of Medical Specialties joint initiative. These competencies include assessment of patient care, interpersonal and communication skills, professionalism, medical knowledge, practice-based learning and improvement, and systems-based practice.

Our policies require completion of the enclosed form. Failure to receive this form will delay consideration of the applicant's request for privileges. Also, our policies require the physician to document competency in performing specific procedures by allowing our organization to obtain a copy of his/her privilege form from your facility as well as a list of the actual procedures performed in the past 12 months and the outcomes (if outcome information is available) for those procedures. The applicant has authorized you to provide this information to our organization via signature on the attached Authorization and Release Form.

Sincerely,

Medical Staff Coordinator

3.8 — Sample Letter Re: Facility Privileges and Competency Validation *(cont.)*

CONFIDENTIAL Evaluation of Facility Privileges and Competency Validation

Name of facility providing information: _____

Name of practitioner for which information is provided: _____

Dates on staff: From _____ To _____

Has the practitioner been subject to any disciplinary action, restrictions, modifications, or loss of privileges or medical staff appointment either voluntary or involuntary at your facility or did the practitioner resign in lieu of such action?   ❑ Yes ❑ No

Are you aware of any restrictions, modifications, or loss of privileges or medical staff appointment, either voluntary or involuntary, at any another facility?   ❑ Yes ❑ No

Are you aware of any physical or mental condition that could affect this practitioner's ability to exercise clinical privileges as requested or that would require accommodation to perform privileges safely and competently?   ❑ Yes ❑ No

If the answer to any of the above questions is "Yes," please explain:

_____

<u>Evaluation:</u>   Please rate the practitioner in the following areas.

- **Patient care** is compassionate, appropriate, and effective for the treatment of health problems and promotion of health
- **Medical knowledge** about established and evolving biomedical, clinical, and cognate (e.g., epidemiological and social-behavioral) sciences and the application of this knowledge to patient care
- **Practice-based learning and improvement** that involves investigation and evaluation of their own patient care, appraisal and assimilation of scientific evidence, and improvements in patient care
- **Interpersonal and communication skills** that result in effective information exchange and teaming with patients, their families, and other health professionals

| 3.8 | Sample Letter Re: Facility Privileges and Competency Validation *(cont.)* |

- **Professionalism,** as manifested through a commitment to carrying out professional responsibilities, adherence to ethical principles, and sensitivity to a diverse patient population
- **Systems-based practice,** as manifested by actions that demonstrate an awareness of and responsiveness to the larger context and system of healthcare and the ability to effectively call on system resources to provide care that is of optimal value

	Excellent	Good	Fair	Poor	Unable to evaluate
Patient care					
Medical knowledge					
Practice-based learning and improvement					
Interpersonal and communication skills					
Professionalism					
Systems-based practice					

This evaluation is based on:

❏ Personal knowledge of the applicant

❏ Review of file

❏ Other _____

_____

_____   _____
Signature   Date

_____   _____
Name, Position/Title (please print)   Phone Number

3.9   Sample Letter for Verification of Training

[Date]

Re: [Applicant's full name, Title]
Training: [Residency/fellowship]
Specialty: [Specialty]
Dates: [From/to]

Dear [Program Director name]:

We have received an application from the above-named provider for medical staff appointment and/or privileges. A copy of the privileges requested is attached. The applicant noted that the above-specified training took place at your institution. In order to process the application, we require verification of completion of training and documentation of experience, ability, and current competence on the six areas of "general competencies" adopted from the Accreditation Council for Graduate Medical Education and the American Board of Medical Specialties joint initiative.

Our policies require completion of the enclosed form. Failure to receive this form will delay consideration of the applicant's request for privileges. Also, our policies require the physician to document competency in performing specific procedures by allowing our organization to obtain a copy of his/her procedure list from your program and the outcomes for those procedures (if outcomes are available). The applicant has authorized you to provide this information to our organization via signature on the attached Authorization and Release Form.

Enclosed is a copy of a release and immunity statement signed by the applicant consenting to this inquiry and your response. The immunity statement releases from liability any individual who provides the requested information.

Thank you for your assistance. We look forward to hearing from you.

Sincerely,

Director

Enclosures

3.9	Sample Letter for Verification of Training *(cont.)*

Residency Program Director's Evaluation and Recommendation

Page 1

Re: [*Applicant's full name*]

Training: [Residency/fellowship]

Specialty: [Specialty]

Dates: [From/to]

	Area of Evaluation *Please use comment section below to provide additional information noting question number for which information is provided.*	YES	NO	Unable to evaluate
1	Were you the director of the program at the time of this applicant's training?			
2	Was the applicant at your institution in the above program for the stated period of time?			
3	Was the program fully accredited throughout the applicant's participation in it?			
4	Did the applicant successfully complete the program?			
5	Did the applicant receive satisfactory ratings for all aspects of his/her training in the program?			
6	Was the applicant ever subject to or considered for disciplinary action?			
7	Did the applicant ever attempt procedures beyond his/her assigned training protocols?			
8	Was the applicant's status and/or authority to provide services ever revoked, suspended, reduced, restricted, not renewed, or was he/she placed on probationary status or reprimanded at any time or were proceedings ever initiated that could have led to any of the actions?			
9	Did the applicant ever voluntarily terminate his/her status in the program or restrict his/her activities in the program in lieu of formal action or to avoid an investigation?			

| 3.9 | Sample Letter for Verification of Training *(cont.)* |

Area of Evaluation *Please use comment section below to provide additional information noting question number for which information is provided.*	YES	NO	Unable to evaluate
10	In reviewing the attached request for privileges, do you feel that the applicant's training and experience included these procedures?			
11	In reviewing the attached request for privileges, do you feel that the applicant is currently competent to carry out these procedures?			
12	Are you aware of any physical or mental condition that could affect this practitioner's ability to exercise clinical privileges in his/her specialty area or that would require an accommodation to exercise those privileges safely and competently?			

Comments:

Question   Comment

_____   _____

_____   _____

_____   _____

_____   _____

_____   _____

_____   _____

_____   _____

_____   _____

_____   _____

_____   _____

| 3.9 | Sample Letter for Verification of Training *(cont.)* |

Residency Program Director's Evaluation and Recommendation
Page 2

Re: [*Applicant's full name*]

Training: [Residency/fellowship]

Specialty: [Specialty]

Dates: [From/to]

Please rate the applicant in each of the following areas:

	Excellent	Good	Fair	Poor	Unable to evaluate
Patient care					
Medical knowledge					
Practice-based learning and improvement					
Interpersonal and communication skills					
Professionalism					
Systems-based practice					

This evaluation is based on:

❑ Personal knowledge of the applicant

❑ Review of file

❑ Other _____

Overall Recommendation (check ONE):

❑ I recommend privileges as requested without reservation.

❑ I recommend privileges as requested with the following reservation(s) (use back of form, if necessary):

_____

_____

3.9	Sample Letter for Verification of Training *(cont.)*

❏ I do not recommend this applicant for the following reason(s):

_____

_____

_____   _____
Signature   Date

_____   _____
Name, Position/Title (please print)   Phone Number

Please return this form within two weeks. Failure to receive the form will delay consideration of the applicant's request for privileges.

The hospital must have a clearly documented procedure for processing requests for initial grants, renewal, or revision of privileges, which must be approved by the medical staff.

The privileging process must include a statement to which the applicant must attest that there are no existing health problems that could affect his or her ability to perform the requested privileges. This statement must be confirmed. For initial applicants, health status can be confirmed by the director of a training program, the chief of services or chief of staff at another hospital at which privileges are currently held, or by a medical staff–approved licensed physician. If there is doubt about an applicant's ability to perform privileges requested, the medical staff has the option of requiring an evaluation by an external and internal source.

The hospital must query the National Practitioner Data Bank (NPDB), as required by law, on initial grants of privileges, renewal of privileges, and when new privileges are requested. This is required by the Health Care Quality Improvement Act.

Before recommending privileges, the medical staff must evaluate each of the bulleted areas noted below:

- Challenges to any licensure or registration

- Voluntary and/or involuntary relinquishment of any license or registration

Note that for the previous two bulleted items, the standard requires evaluation of actions against *any licensure or registration*. This means that all licensure or registration currently or previously held in any state needs to be evaluated for challenges. The Joint Commission allows the use of the FSMB Physician Data Center's services for verification of actions taken against a physician's medical license.

- Voluntary and/or involuntary termination of medical staff membership and voluntary and/or involuntary limitation, reduction, or loss of clinical privileges

- Evidence of an excessive number or an unusual pattern of professional lawsuits that resulted in a final judgment against the applicant

- Documentation as to the applicant's health status

- Relevant practitioner-specific data as compared to aggregate data, when available

- Morbidity and mortality data, when available

The hospital must have a process to determine whether it has adequate clinical performance information to make its decision regarding the granting, limiting, or denial of privileges. This means that there should be a documented process for determining whether there is enough information to make a privileging decision.

Action taken on requests for privileges must be made within a time period that is specified in the medical staff bylaws. This is one of the few EPs in the Medical Staff chapter that is scored as a "C." This EP also contains an "M" icon, meaning that a "measure of success" will be necessary if the hospital is found to be noncompliant. Compliance is based on the frequency with which the EP is not met. Each time an area of noncompliance is identified, it is counted as a separate occurrence. For example, if the surveyor reviews a sample of 20 credentials files and finds that three are not processed within the required time frame, each one is counted as a separate occurrence.

When changes in clinical privileges are made, information regarding the practitioner's scope of privileges is updated. Privilege forms in credentials files and any reference to privileges throughout the organization must be updated. Affected hospital departments must be notified of changes. (See also MS.06.01.09.)

The Joint Commission defines "peer recommendation" as "information submitted by a practitioner in the same professional discipline as the applicant reflecting the practitioner's perception of the applicant's clinical practice, ability to work as part of a team, and ethical behavior or the documented peer evaluation of practitioner-specific data collected from various sources for the purpose of evaluating current competence." A physician must provide the peer recommendation for a physician, dentist for dentist, podiatrist for podiatrist, nurse for nurse, etc.

Peer recommendations must be obtained from a practitioner in the same professional discipline as the applicant with personal knowledge of the applicant's ability to practice and must include information regarding the following:

- **Medical/clinical knowledge.** Practitioners should have a good working knowledge of established and evolving biomedical, clinical, and cognate sciences, and how to apply this knowledge to patient care. This is evidenced by completion of educational and training requirements, as well as by on-the-job experience, in-service training, and continuing education.

- **Technical and clinical skills.** Skill involves the capacity to perform specific privileges/procedures. It is based on both knowledge and the ability to apply that knowledge. Skills can be gained by hands-on training using anatomic models or real patients. For instance, a surgeon learning to use a laser may use animal tissue in hands-on training rather than a human subject.

- **Clinical judgment.** Clinical judgment refers to the observations, perceptions, impressions, recollections, intuitions, beliefs, feelings, and inferences of providers. These clinical judgments are used to reach decisions, individually or collectively with other providers, about a patient's diagnosis and treatment. It comes into play on a daily basis.

- **Interpersonal skills.** Areas of evaluation include how the provider works effectively with other professional associates, including those from other disciplines, to provide patient-focused care as a member of a healthcare team.

- **Communication skills.** The provider should create and sustain a therapeutic and ethically sound relationship with other caregivers, patients, and their families. He or she should be able to communicate effectively and demonstrate caring, compassionate, and respectful behavior. This includes effective listening skills, effective nonverbal communication, the ability to elicit/provide information, and good writing skills.

- **Professionalism.** Professionalism is demonstrated by respect, compassion, and integrity. It means being responsive and accountable to the needs of the patient, society, and the profession. It also means being committed to providing high-quality patient care and continuous professional development, as well as being ethical in issues related to clinical care, patient confidentiality, informed consent, and business practices.

There are additional requirements in MS.07.01.03 for peer recommendations. For the benefit of flow, we are including these here.

MS.07.01.03: Peer recommendations

The medical staff must use peer recommendations in its consideration of recommendations for appointment and initial granting of privileges, as well as in consideration of termination from the medical staff or revision/revocation of clinical privileges. Peers should be knowledgeable about the applicant's professional performance and competence. Examples of appropriate sources for peer recommendations include: a PI committee with a majority of members who are peers, reference letters, documented telephone conversations, department or service chair, or the MEC.

If there are insufficient practitioner-specific data available when the medical staff is renewing privileges, the medical staff uses and evaluates peer recommendations. Note that peer recommendations are only required at reappointment if there is insufficient data to support the continuation of privileges. This standard is not meant to imply that peer recommendations can substitute for ongoing professional practice evaluation.

The letter in Figure 3.10, Sample Peer Recommendation Letter, can be used for documenting peer recommendations.

3.10	Sample Peer Recommendation Letter

Date

Facility Name

Facility Address

Regarding applicant: John Doe, MD

Specialty: General Surgery

Dear _____:

We have received an application from the above-named provider for medical staff appointment and privileges. A copy of the privileges requested is attached. The applicant has listed you as a peer who will be willing to provide a recommendation. In order to process the application, we require your evaluation of the applicant's experience, ability, and current competence in the areas of medical/clinical knowledge, technical and clinical skills, clinical judgment, interpersonal skills, communication skills, and professionalism.

Our policies require completion of the enclosed form. Failure to receive this form will delay consideration of the applicant's request for privileges. You may supplement the form with additional information, if you so desire. The applicant has authorized you to provide this information to our organization via signature on the attached Authorization and Release Form.

Sincerely,

Medical Staff Coordinator

3.10 Sample Peer Recommendation Letter *(cont.)*

CONFIDENTIAL Professional Peer Reference & Competency Validation
Page 1 of 2

Name of Applicant: _____

Name of Evaluator: _____ Relationship to Applicant: _____

How well do you know the applicant?　　❑ Not well　　　　　　❑ Casual personal acquaintance

　　　　　　　　　　　　　　　　　❑ Professional acquaintance　❑ Very well

Do you refer your patients to the applicant?　　❑ Yes　　❑ No

If no, list reason(s) why not _____

_____

PLEASE RATE THE PRACTITIONER IN THE FOLLOWING AREAS

	Excellent	Good	Fair	Poor	Unable to evaluate
Medical knowledge: Practitioner should have a good working knowledge of established and evolving biomedical, clinical, and cognate sciences and how to apply this knowledge to patient care. This is evidenced by completion of educational and training requirements as well as on-the-job experience, in-service training, and continuing education.					
Technical and clinical skills: Skill involves the capacity to perform specific privileges/procedures. It is based on both knowledge and the ability to apply that knowledge.					

3.10	Sample Peer Recommendation Letter *(cont.)*

	Excellent	Good	Fair	Poor	Unable to evaluate
Clinical judgment: Clinical judgment refers to the observations, perceptions, impressions, recollections, intuitions, beliefs, feelings, and inferences of providers. These clinical judgments are used to reach decisions, individually and/or collectively with other providers, about a patient's diagnosis and treatment.					
Communication skills: The provider should create and sustain a therapeutic and ethically sound relationship with other caregivers, patients, and their families. He/she should be able to communicate effectively and demonstrates caring, compassionate, and respectful behavior. This also includes effective listening skills, effective nonverbal communication, eliciting/providing information, and good writing skills.					
Interpersonal skills: Areas of evaluation include how the provider works effectively with other professional associates, including those from other disciplines, to provide patient-focused care as a member of a healthcare team.					
Professionalism: Professionalism is demonstrated by respect, compassion, and integrity. It means being responsive and accountable to the needs of the patient, society, and the profession. It also means being committed to providing high-quality patient care and continuous professional development as well as being ethical in issues related to clinical care, patient confidentiality, informed consent, and business practices.					

3.10   Sample Peer Recommendation Letter *(cont.)*

CONFIDENTIAL Professional Peer Reference & Competency Validation
Page 2 of 2

Name of Applicant:_____

Name of Evaluator:_____

Relevant training and experience: In reviewing the attached request for privileges, do you feel that the applicant's training and experience are adequate to carry out these procedures?

❑ No—If no, please provide an explanation _____

❑ Yes

❑ Unable to evaluate

Current competence: In reviewing the attached request for privileges, do you feel that the applicant is currently competent to carry out these procedures?

❑ No—If no, please provide an explanation _____

❑ Yes

❑ Unable to evaluate

Health Status: Are you aware of any physical or mental condition that could affect this practitioner's ability to exercise clinical privileges in his/her specialty area or that would require an accommodation to exercise those privileges safely and competently?

❑ No

❑ Yes—If yes, please provide an explanation _____

❑ Unable to evaluate

3.10	Sample Peer Recommendation Letter *(cont.)*

Overall Recommendation (check ONE):

❑ I recommend privileges as requested without reservation.

❑ I recommend privileges as requested with the following reservation(s) (use back of form, if necessary):

_____

_____

❑ I do not recommend this applicant for the following reason(s):

_____

_____

_____	_____
Signature	Date

_____	_____
Name, Position/Title (please print)	Phone Number

Please return this form within two weeks. Failure to receive the form will delay consideration of the applicant's request for privileges.

MS.06.01.07: Analysis and use of information received

This standard requires the medical staff to actually review and analyze the information collected by the hospital during the credentialing and privileging process and use it to come to its decisions. The process used for review and analysis of information must be clearly defined. This will require a written, documented process. Information reviewed must include current licensure status, training, experience, current competence, and ability to perform the requested privileges. Whatever process the hospital uses for making credentialing and privileging decisions, it must ensure that decisions are made in a timely manner. If your hospital is having problems with processing applications or reapplications within the required time frames, it may be helpful to use a tracking form such as the one in Figure 3.11 for analyzing delays in the process.

3.11 — Tracking Form for New Applications and Reapplications [Hospital Name] Medical Staff

Name of Applicant	Department	Application Type	Date Returned	Date Completed*	Days to Complete*	Date Chair Review	Days to Complete Chair Review	Date Credential Committee Recommendation	Days to Complete Credential Com. Recommendation	Date MEC Recommendation	Days to Complete MEC Review	Date Board Action	Days to Complete Board Review/Action	Total Days From Completion to Action
AVERAGES														

*A complete application is one in which the application itself is not only complete, but all primary source verification and information required by the medical staff bylaws is completed.

The organization develops the criteria that will be used in the decision to grant, limit, or deny a requested privilege. Gender, race, creed, or national origin cannot be factored into decisions regarding medical staff membership. Criteria are based on recommendations of the medical staff and are approved by the governing body. Criteria must be consistently applied to all practitioners.

Criteria used to make decisions on medical staff membership and clinical privileges must be directly related to the quality of healthcare, treatment, and services. If privileging criteria are used that are unrelated to quality of care, treatment, and services or professional competence, evidence must exist that the effect of resulting decisions on the quality of care, treatment, and services is evaluated.

Privileges are granted for a period not to exceed two years. Reappointments must be made no later than two years from the date of the previous appointment. To accomplish this goal, the governing body should approve applications in advance of the expiration date with a designated effective date. For instance, if privileges and appointment expire January 1, the board should take action prior to that date and appoint with an effective date of January 1.

Final authority for granting, renewing, or denying privileges rests with the governing body or a committee to which the governing body has delegated this function. MS.06.01.11 includes some additional requirements regarding this option for delegation.

MS.06.01.11: Expedited credentialing

An expedited process for appointment/reappointment and privileges can be used by the organization. Although this is addressed in the medical staff standards, the expedited approval process is actually a function of the governing body.

The Joint Commission allows expedited credentialing by enabling the governing body to delegate appointment and privileging decisions to a committee consisting of at least two voting governing body members. The MEC function cannot be delegated; only the board function can be delegated. Some refer to this process as "fast-track" credentialing.

MS.01.01.01 requires the medical staff bylaws to document the credentialing process, including temporary and disaster privileges, but it does not specifically address including the criteria for expedited credentialing in the medical staff bylaws. Because other credentialing criteria are required to be in the bylaws, however, the criteria for expediting should also be included there.

The medical staff develops the criteria for an expedited process, and these criteria must be appropriately followed. Criteria must state that expedited credentialing may not be used if the applicant's application is incomplete or the MEC makes a final recommendation that is adverse or has limitations.

The standards list situations that should be evaluated on a case-by-case basis and that would usually lead to ineligibility for expedited credentialing, including:

- There is a current challenge or a previously successful challenge to licensure or registration

- There has been an involuntary termination of medical staff membership or an involuntary limitation, reduction, denial, or loss of clinical privileges at another organization

- There is an unusual pattern or an excessive number of professional liability actions that resulted in a final judgment against the applicant

This standard does not say that these issues definitely make the practitioner ineligible, only that they must be evaluated on a case-by-case basis. It is up to the organization to decide whether to grant the privileges after a thorough evaluation of the particular incident.

If all committees are meeting on a regular basis and there are no delays in processing applications in a timely manner, your organization may not need to use an expedited process. If your board meets infrequently, however, it may be appropriate to consider an expedited credentialing approval process. See Figure 3.12 for a sample policy and procedure.

| 3.12 | Sample Medical Staff Expedited Credentialing Policy and Procedure |

PURPOSE:

This policy and procedure is made for rendering appointment, reappointment, and privileging decisions through an expedited credentialing process without compromising the quality of the review. "Expedited credentialing" provides an expedited review and approval process if specific, predefined criteria are met.

Expedited credentialing is neither a right nor a privilege. Candidates who do not meet the criteria for expedited credentialing will be processed through the usual credentialing process as specified in the medical staff bylaws.

PROCEDURE:

The department chair and medical staff coordinator, or their designee(s), will review each application, its associated documentation, and the information acquired during the credentialing and privileging process to determine eligibility.

In order to be eligible for expedited approval, the criteria in 1–9 must be met:

1. The application is complete and accurate with all requested information returned. (A complete application is one in which not only the application is complete, but all primary source verification and information required by the medical staff bylaws is completed.)

2. There are no discrepancies in information received and no negative or questionable information is received.

3. Medical staff/work history is unremarkable (e.g., no frequent moves, unexplained or alarming gaps).

4. The applicant's request for clinical privileges is consistent with the medical staff's designation for applicant's specialty, his/her experience, training, and current competency; and all applicable privileging criteria are met.

5. The applicant possesses a current, valid state license, professional liability insurance in limits specified by the medical staff, and federal and/or state narcotics certificate(s), if applicable.

3.12	**Sample Medical Staff Expedited Credentialing Policy and Procedure** *(cont.)*

6. The applicant has indicated that he/she can safely and competently exercise the clinical privileges requested, with or without a reasonable accommodation.

7. The applicant's history shows an ability to relate to others in a harmonious, collegial manner.

8. At the time of renewal of privileges, documentation of activity in the hospital and/or verification from outside healthcare entities and/or peers sufficiently verifies current competence.

9. At the time of renewal of privileges, the results of peer review activities and the quality improvement functions of the medical staff reveal no areas of concern.

Each of the criteria in 10–16 below will be thoroughly evaluated on a case-by-case basis and may lead to ineligibility for expedited credentialing:

10. The applicant's medical staff appointment, staff status, and/or clinical privileges have never been involuntarily resigned, denied, revoked, suspended, restricted, reduced, surrendered, or not renewed at any other healthcare facility.

11. The applicant has never withdrawn application for appointment, reappointment, or clinical privileges or resigned from the medical staff before a decision was made by another healthcare facility's governing board or in order to avoid denial or termination of such.

12. No license(s), DEA or other controlled-substance authorizations, membership in local, state, or national professional societies, or board certification have ever been suspended, modified, terminated, or voluntarily or involuntarily surrendered.

13. The applicant has not been named as a defendant in a criminal action and/or has not been convicted of a crime.

14. There are no significant adverse findings reported by the National Practitioner Data Bank, Healthcare Practitioner Data Bank, Federation of State Medical Boards, the AMA/American Osteopathic Association, or any other practitioner database.

<table>
<tr><td>3.12</td><td>Sample Medical Staff Expedited Credentialing
Policy and Procedure *(cont.)*</td></tr>
</table>

15. There are no past or pending malpractice actions, including claims, lawsuits, arbitrations, settlements, awards, or judgments, that show an unusual pattern or an excessive number of professional liability actions resulting in a final judgment against the applicant.

16. There are no proposed or actual exclusions and/or any pending investigations of the applicant from any healthcare program funded in whole or in part by the federal government, including Medicare or Medicaid.

Processing of applications:

1. The medical staff office receives and processes the application according to organization and medical staff policy.

   If, at any point in the process below, any reviewer feels the application does not meet criteria for expedited credentialing, the file will be processed and transmitted through the full review process as outlined in the medical staff bylaws.

2. The appropriate department chair or designee reviews the completed and verified application and forwards a report with findings and a recommendation to the medical executive committee.

3. The medical executive committee reviews the application at its next scheduled meeting and forwards its recommendation to the governing body's credentials committee.

4. The governing body's credentials committee reviews and evaluates the qualifications and competence of the practitioner applying for appointment, reappointment, or renewal or modification of clinical privileges and renders its decision. A positive decision results in the appointment or privileges requested. The date of the committee's decision is the approval date, or the committee may assign an "effective" approval date.

   If the decision is adverse to an applicant, the matter will be referred back to the medical staff executive committee for further evaluation.

   The governing body's credentials committee will report its recommendation to the full board.

MS.06.01.09: Privilege decision notification

Decisions regarding granting, limiting, revoking, or denying existing or renewal of privileges must be communicated to the practitioner within the time frame specified in the medical staff bylaws.

If privileges are denied, the applicant must be informed of the reason. When adverse decisions are made, the organization must make the practitioner aware of any available due process or, if applicable, the option to implement the fair hearing and appeal process.

The decision to grant, deny, revise, or revoke privileges is distributed and made available to all appropriate internal persons and to all external persons or entities, as delineated by the organization and as required by law. Hospitals should ensure that appropriate hospital patient care areas/departments are informed of the privileges granted to the practitioner or any revisions or revocations. Medical staff leaders, such as the MEC and department chairs, should be notified, particularly if the board's decision differs from the MEC's recommendations. Whenever a practitioner's privileges are limited, revoked, or in any way constrained, the hospital must report those constraints to appropriate state and federal authorities, registries, and databases, such as the NPDB.

The medical staff must approve the process used to distribute information regarding the decision to grant, deny, revise, or revoke privileges. This EP contains a "D" icon, meaning the surveyor will be looking for documentation to determine compliance. Check to be sure that the hospital has a written procedure for distributing information to internal and external sources and documentation of the medical staff's (or MEC's) approval of the process. Figure 3.13 is a sample Policy for Notification of Internal and External Parties Regarding Practitioner Privileges. This policy is included on the Tools website.

3.13	Notification of Internal and External Parties Regarding Practitioner Privileges

Policy:

Key external and internal persons and organizations must be notified whenever a change occurs in a practitioner's privileges or when a new practitioner is granted privileges or appointment. Some internal sources require information regarding clinical privileges granted, whereas others require only a general notification.

Procedure:

Internal Sources:

General Notification of New Practitioner:

When a new practitioner is granted medical staff appointment or clinical privileges, a general notification should be distributed via e-mail or memo to all hospital departments. The following information should be included:

Full name
- Credentials
- Address
- Phone
- Fax
- Pager/paging service number
- Partners, alternates
- Effective date
- Picture
- Sponsoring physician (if AHP)

3.13	Notification of Internal and External Parties Regarding Practitioner Privileges *(cont.)*

General Notification Practitioner Leaving Staff:

When a practitioner leaves the staff, a general notification should be distributed via e-mail or memo to all hospital departments. The following information should be included:

- Full name
- Credential
- Forwarding address (if applicable)
- Effective date

Notification of Privileges

When new privileges are granted either to a new applicant or an existing medical staff member or allied health professional, or when there is a modification (addition, deletion, termination, proctorship, etc.) to current privileges, the following internal personnel should be notified via e-mail or memo, and a copy of the privileges (or modification to privileges) should be included with the notification. *(Note: Will need to modify this language to reference privileges that are posted via intranet or other electronic means.)*

[Name]   Admitting department

[Name]   Operating room

[Name]   Nursing administration (for distribution to all nursing units)

[Name]   Administration

[Name]   Emergency department

[Name]   Outpatient/ambulatory clinic(s)

[Name]   Quality management

[Name]   *(Include others, as appropriate)*

| 3.13 | **Notification of Internal and External Parties Regarding Practitioner Privileges** *(cont.)* |

External Sources

National Practitioner Data Bank and State Licensing Boards

The Health Care Quality Improvement Act of 1986 includes a requirement for reporting of certain adverse actions to the National Practitioner Data Bank.

Hospitals must report:

(1) A professional review action that adversely affects a physician's or dentist's clinical privileges for more than 30 days and is based on the physician's or dentist's professional competence or professional conduct; and

(2) The voluntary surrender of clinical privileges by a physician or dentist who is under investigation relating to questions of professional competence or conduct, or in return for no investigation or professional review action being conducted.

A professional review action includes denying, reducing, restricting, revoking, and suspending privileges, and also includes a decision not to renew clinical privileges if that action is based on the physician's or dentist's professional competence or conduct.

Hospitals must submit adverse action reports to the appropriate state licensing board within 15 days of final board action in the case of an adverse action or within 15 days of the date the physician surrenders his or her clinical privileges. These reports must be submitted electronically to the National Practitioner Data Bank as an Adverse Action Report. Within 15 days, a printed copy of the electronic report must be forwarded to the state medical licensing board.

Revisions to previously reported adverse actions must also be reported. For example, if a physician's clinical privileges are reinstated after a 45-day suspension, both the suspension and the reinstatement must be reported.

Note: All reports to state licensing boards and the NPDB should be coordinated with the legal department.

MS.06.01.13: Temporary privileges

In certain circumstances, standards allow the CEO, or his or her authorized designee, to grant temporary privileges for a limited time period. This must be done only on the recommendation of the medical staff president or his or her authorized designee. The Joint Commission allows two circumstances for which the granting of temporary privileges to an LIP would be acceptable: to fulfill an important patient care need, and when a new applicant with a complete application that raises no concerns is awaiting review and approval of the MEC and board.

The time period for granting privileges to meet an important care need must be defined in the medical staff bylaws. The organization can define the type of need (e.g., a required skill, a required number of practitioners to cover in the absence of a practitioner). If the hospital perceives a patient need on a service level (e.g., if there are not enough emergency physicians to staff the emergency department in a safe, quality manner), a patient care need can be established. In the case of granting temporary privileges to meet an important patient care need, standards require verification of current licensure and current competence prior to granting privileges. This means that there must be feedback from someone who can make substantive comments regarding the practitioner's ability to perform the requested privileges or data that show competency.

Temporary privileges may be granted for new applicants with a complete application who are awaiting medical staff review and approval for a period that does not exceed 120 days. First, verification of current licensure, relevant training or experience, current competence, ability to perform the privileges requested, and evaluation of NPDB query must be accomplished. In addition, there must not be any current or previously successful challenges to licensure or registration and no involuntary termination of medical staff membership or involuntary limitation, reduction, denial, or loss of clinical privileges at another organization.

See Figure 3.14 for sample bylaws language for temporary privileges.

3.14   Sample Bylaws Language for Temporary Privileges

Temporary privileges may be granted by the hospital CEO or authorized designee on recommendation of the medical staff president or authorized designee in the following circumstances:

Patient care need. In the case of a circumstance in which privileges are required to fulfill a patient care need, temporary privileges may be granted upon written request of the practitioner. Types of patient care needs include: the need for a practitioner who has a required skill, a required number of practitioners to adequately cover a service, and to provide coverage in the absence of a practitioner. The time limit for privileges will be considered on a case-by-case basis but will not exceed 60 days. Prior to granting of such privileges, documentation of the patient care need, verification of current licensure, current competency, and National Practitioner Data Bank (NPDB) query will be obtained and evaluated.

New applicants. Upon receipt of a complete application (as defined by the medical staff) for medical staff appointment and a written request for temporary privileges, temporary privileges may be granted for a period not to exceed 120 days while awaiting approval of the application. In order to be eligible for temporary privileges, there must be no evidence of a current or previously successful challenge to licensure or registration, involuntary termination of medical staff membership at another organization, or involuntary limitation, reduction, denial, or loss of clinical privileges. Prior to granting temporary privileges, verification of the following must be obtained and evaluated:

- Current licensure
- Relevant training or experience
- Current competence
- Ability to perform the privileges requested
- NPDB query

In addition, the following criteria must be met:

- No health concerns regarding the privileges requested
- Appropriate alternative coverage
- Meets criteria for privileges
- Adequate professional liability insurance
- CME requirements

MS.07.01.01: Medical staff appointment

The medical staff makes recommendations to the governing body for medical staff appointment as part of its oversight of the quality of care, treatment, and services provided by privileged practitioners. The medical staff does not approve, but only recommends. The governing body is the final authority that makes the decision on whether to appoint the practitioner.

The medical staff develops criteria for medical staff membership and uses these criteria in appointing its members. Criteria should be designed to assure the medical staff and governing body that patients will receive quality care, treatment, and services. MS.01.01.01 requires that these criteria be spelled out in the medical staff bylaws. Examples of appointment criteria include state licensure, professional liability insurance with specific limits, education, training, and office and residence located within a specific geographic area.

Appointments to the medical staff, like clinical privileges, cannot exceed a period of two years. Gender, race, creed, or national origin cannot be factored into privileging decisions.

MS.08.01.01: Focused professional practice evaluation

According to The Joint Commission, focused professional practice evaluation (FPPE) applies to a practitioner for which the hospital does not have documented evidence of competently performing the requested privileges at the organization. It also can apply when a question arises concerning the ability of a practitioner with current privileges to provide safe, high-quality patient care.

FPPE must be consistently implemented according to the medical staff's criteria and requirements. All initially requested privileges are subject to a period of FPPE. Circumstances that require monitoring and evaluation of a practitioner's professional performance must be defined by the medical staff. In addition, the medical staff develops criteria for evaluating the performance of practitioners credentialed and privileged through the medical staff process when a question about whether safe, high-quality patient care is identified. For instance, if the credentialing and privileging processes show that a provider has not performed a sufficient number of procedures so that the medical staff is comfortable with granting full, unrestricted privileges, the organization may require a certain number of procedures to be granted under proctorship. Another example is that if a currently privileged provider's performance is not consistent with what the medical staff feels is high-quality care, criteria for focused monitoring for that specific practitioner may include 100% monitoring of all cases.

The documented performance monitoring process includes the following:

- The criteria to be used for performance monitoring. Potential criteria may include reviewing patient medical records, evaluating clinical practice patterns, proctoring for specific procedures or for overall care provided, and conducting general discussion with other individuals involved in the care of each patient.

- The method used for establishing a monitoring plan specific to the requested privilege. The medical staff may develop separate monitoring processes depending on the privileges requested. Retrospective or concurrent review—or a combination of both— may be conducted. This could vary depending on the privileges requested and the specialty of the provider. A surgeon or physician performing high-risk surgical or interventional procedures may be assigned a proctor who will show up in the operating room and observe a certain number of procedures. A family practice physician who does not perform any procedures may have patient charts reviewed either while the patient is in-house or retrospectively, on discharge.

- The method used for determining how long the performance monitoring will last. The methods used should not be based on arbitrary criteria, such as random number of procedures performed, but should be scientifically developed, consensus driven, and based on current literature. For instance, the Heart Rhythm Society's Clinical Competency Statement: Training Pathways for Implantation of Cardioverter Defibrillators and Cardiac Resynchronization Devices provides the minimum competency standards for physicians implanting cardioverter defibrillators or cardiac resynchronization therapy devices. An addendum to this clinical competency statement defines proctoring requirements for these procedures.

- Circumstances requiring monitoring to be conducted by an external source must be defined. There may be times when no one on the medical staff can provide monitoring. There may not be anyone who has the specific privileges, or those who do have them may have a conflict of interest. In these cases, the organization should seek an outside source for monitoring. This can be accomplished through having a proctor come to the facility to review a procedure, through retrospective review of medical records, or, in the case of diagnostic imaging, films can be sent to outside reviewers for an over-read.

The medical staff's FPPE plan must identify any triggers that would indicate the need for performance monitoring. Triggers can be a single event, such as a surgical incident involving death or serious adverse outcome, or a negative clinical practice trend identified through the organization's PI activities.

Decisions to perform focused professional performance monitoring to further assess current competence must be based on the evaluation of a practitioner's current clinical competence, practice behavior, and ability to perform the requested privilege.

The medical staff develops criteria to determine the type of monitoring to be conducted. The monitoring process may vary depending on the type of provider and the event being monitored. A practitioner may be assigned a focused review for a certain surgical procedure or set of privileges, or it may be assigned a focused period for all requested privileges. The organization clearly delineates the measures employed in resolving performance issues, and these measures must be consistently implemented. Examples of measures taken to resolve performance issues include a documented discussion with the practitioner by the department chair, a letter to the provider noting areas in need of improvement, recommendations for training, focused monitoring, and subsequent corrective action. When issues are identified, communication to the provider must be clear and specific about what is wrong with the performance and what improvements are expected.

In reporting the results of FPPE, your medical staff may wish to utilize a form, such as that in Figure 3.15. This form is included on the Tools website.

3.15   Sample Form for Documentation of FPPE Results

Name of practitioner: _____

Data reviewed for the following dates   From: _____ To: _____

Based on the review and evaluation of information resulting from the focused professional practice evaluation, the following recommendation(s) are made:

❑ Practitioner is performing well or within desired expectations and no further focused review is necessary.

❑ The practitioner has not provided an adequate volume of patient care or treatment in order to render an opinion. FPPE to continue for _____ (e.g., three months, six months)

❑ Practitioner is NOT performing well or within desired expectations and further action is recommended.

     ❑ Focused evaluation to continue. (List issue[s].)

     _____

     _____

     ❑ There is the possibility of risk to patient safety and it is recommended that privileges be suspended.

     ❑ Other (List)

     _____

     _____

_____   _____
Signature of Reviewer   Date

_____
Title of Reviewer

MS.08.01.03: Ongoing professional practice evaluation

Ongoing professional practice evaluation (OPPE) is the process that the hospital and medical staff use to identify negative practice trends that may affect quality of care and patient safety. Prior to or at the time of renewal/reappointment of privileges, information collected as a result of the organization's OPPE is used in the decision to maintain current privileges or to revise/revoke an existing privilege.

A clearly defined process must be in effect, and the process must facilitate evaluation of the professional practice of each practitioner. Individual medical staff departments determine what performance data to collect. This is then approved by the organized medical staff. The medical staff uses the information it receives from OPPE in its determination whether to continue, limit, or revoke any existing privileges.

In reporting the results of OPPE, your medical staff may wish to utilize a form, such as that in Figure 3.16.

3.16   Sample Form for Documentation of OPPE Results

Name of practitioner: _____

Data reviewed for the following dates: From: _____ To: _____

Based on the review and evaluation of information resulting from the ongoing professional practice evaluation, the following recommendation(s) are made:

❏ Practitioner is performing well or within desired expectations and no further action is warranted.

❏ Practitioner is NOT performing well or within desired expectations and further action is recommended.

    ❏ An issue exists that requires a focused evaluation. (List issue[s].)

    _____

    _____

    ❏ There is the possibility of risk to patient safety and privileges are suspended.

❏ There is not adequate data available to determine whether privileges should continue. The following recommendation(s) is (are) made:

    ❏ Implement a focused review whenever the practitioner actually provides patient care/treatment/services. (See FPPE policy.)

    ❏ Request procedure lists and outcomes from other facilities where the provider is currently providing patient care/treatment/services.

_____   _____
       Signature of Reviewer   Date

_____
       Title of Reviewer

MS.09.01.01: Evaluation and action regarding practitioner-specific concerns

Pursuant to its bylaws, the medical staff evaluates and acts on reported concerns regarding the clinical practice or competence of a privileged practitioner. The organization clearly defines the process used for collecting, investigating, and addressing clinical practice concerns regarding privileged practitioners. This process is based on recommendations by the medical staff and approval of the governing body.

As required by the organization and any applicable laws or regulations, the medical staff consistently investigates and addresses reported concerns regarding the professional practice of a privileged practitioner. Standards in the Rights and Responsibilities of the Individual chapter require the hospital to respond to, review, and, when possible, resolve complaints from patients or their families.

MS.4.50: Fair hearing and appeal process

There must be mechanisms for a fair hearing and appeal process to address adverse decisions regarding reappointment, denial, reduction, suspension, or revocation of privileges that may relate to quality of care, treatment, and services issues. The standard does not state that all adverse decisions should trigger the fair hearing process—only those that relate to quality of care, treatment, and services issues. Automatic suspensions for issues such as failing to complete medical records and not completing applications on time need not trigger a hearing or appeal. Likewise, denials of initial grants of medical staff membership or privileges do not require a hearing under The Joint Commission's standards.

The mechanisms must allow the affected individual a fair opportunity for defense of the alleged wrongs to an unbiased hearing body of the medical staff. There also must be a mechanism by which to appeal the decision of the hearing body to the governing body. The fair hearing and appeal process must be fair. The process may differ for members and nonmembers of the medical staff. That is, an alternative hearing and appeal process may be designated for those LIPs who are granted privileges but not medical staff appointment. There must be a mechanism used to schedule a hearing and procedures for the hearing to follow. The process must specify that the hearing committee will be composed of impartial peers. Anyone in economic competition with the affected individual and anyone who has participated in making the adverse recommendation should not participate as a member of the committee or in the committee's deliberations. As specified in the medical staff bylaws, in conjunction with the governing body, the fair hearing process must provide a mechanism to appeal adverse decisions.

MS.11.01.01: Licensed independent practitioner health

The American Medical Association (AMA) defines the impaired physician as "one who is unable to practice medicine with reasonable skill and safety to patients because of physical or mental illness, including deterioration through the aging process or loss of motor skill, or excessive use or abuse of drugs including alcohol."

The AMA's Code of Ethics states that a physician shall "strive to report physicians deficient in character or competence, or engaging in fraud or deception, to appropriate entities."

Whenever anyone witnesses "suspicious behavior" from a colleague, he or she should report it immediately according to the process specified in the medical staff's or hospital's policies.

Hospital and medical staff policies should include whom to report to and assure the informant that his or her identity will be kept confidential.

The medical staff must create and implement a process to identify and manage health matters of LIPs. This process must be a separate from the disciplinary action process.

The process includes education of LIPs and organization staff regarding recognizing illness and impairment issues specific to LIPs. The standard requires specific training regarding recognizing and dealing with impairment, including defining "at-risk" behaviors.

The policy should include a mechanism for LIPs to refer themselves to the program as well as referral by others while maintaining the confidentiality of the informant. It should also include referral of the LIP to appropriate professional resources for evaluation, diagnosis, and treatment of the condition or concern. The referral resources can be internal or external.

Maintaining the confidentiality of the LIP who is seeking referral or who is being referred for assistance is essential. The exception to this is when applicable law, ethical obligation, or the health and safety of a patient is threatened; in these cases, reports need to be made.

The process must include evaluation of the credibility of a complaint, allegation, or concern made against an LIP. See MS.09.01.01 for more information regarding evaluation and action regarding practitioner-specific concerns.

There must be a process for monitoring the LIP and the safety of patients until the LIP completes rehabilitation and during any required period afterward. The process must allow for reporting to medical staff leadership any occasions in which an LIP is providing treatment in an unsafe manner. One of the primary functions of the medical staff is to provide oversight for the quality of care, treatment, and services provided by practitioners with privileges. Regardless of confidentiality issues, the medical staff leadership needs to be made aware when there is any question regarding the practitioner's ability to provide patient care, treatment, or services in a safe manner.

The process must allow for appropriate actions to be taken when an LIP fails to complete a required rehabilitation program. This process may include summary suspension of privileges or termination of medical staff membership and privileges.

MS.12.01.01: CME

All LIPs and other practitioners privileged through the medical staff process must participate in continuing education (CE). This participation must be documented and decisions on reappointment or renewal/revision of privileges must consider the LIP's participation in CE activities.

The medical staff prioritizes hospital-sponsored educational activities. CE activities offered at the hospital correspond to the type and nature of care, treatment, and services offered by the hospital. For example, if the hospital is a pediatric hospital, it may bring in a pediatric specialist to discuss a new pediatric surgical procedure that is going to be performed at the hospital. The organization uses the results of PI activities in helping to determine what CE topics will be offered. The medical staff should examine its PI activities on a regular basis to determine what kinds of educational offerings could benefit patient care. In fact, the results of specific studies performed by the medical staff can be the topic of the CE activity.

MS.13.01.01: Telemedicine privileges

At the time of this publication, The Joint Commission published changes to the telemedicine standards that were required in order to comply with CMS' *Conditions of Participation* for hospitals. At the time of publication, CMS is reviewing comments to proposed changes in the *Conditions of Participation.*

The section below includes the approved standards at the time of publication, but there may be more changes in Joint Commission standards if CMS revises its regulations based on comments received. The following Joint Commission standard is effective as of March 2011.

The Joint Commission has separate standards for the originating sites and some standards that apply to both distant and originating sites. In addition, some standards apply only to hospitals that use Joint Commission accreditation for deemed status purposes.

Telemedicine standards for originating site only

For hospitals that use Joint Commission accreditation for deemed status purposes, the hospital must credential and privilege all LIP telemedicine providers responsible for the patient's care, treatment, and services via a telemedicine link according to processes specified in standards MS.06.01.03 through MS.06.01.13. If the hospital is using the services of a Medicare-participating hospital for telemedicine services, it can use a copy of the distant site's credentialing packet for privileging. This packet needs to include the privileges granted by the distant site. The distant site must sign attestation confirming that the credentialing packet is complete, accurate, and up-to-date.

If the hospital does not use Joint Commission accreditation for deemed status purposes, LIPs providing care, treatment, and services of a patient via telemedicine link can be credentialed through one of the following three ways:

- The originating site can fully privilege and credential the practitioner according to The Joint Commission's credentialing and privileging standards as specified in the medical staff standards (MS.06.01.03 through MS.06.01.13), the same as it does any LIP who would apply for privileges.

- The practitioner may be privileged at the originating site using credentialing information from the distant site if the distant site is a Joint Commission–accredited organization.

- The originating site can use the credentialing and privileging decision from the distant site if all of the following requirements are met:

  1. The distant site is a hospital or ambulatory care organization accredited by The Joint Commission.

  2. The practitioner has obtained privileges at the distant site for the services to be provided at the originating site.

  3. The originating site provides the distant site practitioner-specific privilege and performance information that can be used to assess the practitioner's quality of care, treatment, and services. This information should include any adverse outcomes related to sentinel events resulting from telemedicine services that meet

The Joint Commission's definition of a reviewable sentinel event. It also should include any complaints about the LIP from patients, other LIPs, or staff at the originating site. When sharing this information, follow confidentiality practices.

MS.13.01.03: Telemedicine standards for both originating and distant sites

The medical staffs at both the originating and distant sites must recommend which patient care, treatment, and services are to be provided by LIPs through a telemedicine link at their individual sites. Surveyors will be looking for written documentation of the medical staff's recommendations regarding telemedicine services, such as those contained in the minutes of the MEC. The clinical services offered must be consistent with commonly accepted quality standards. The American Telemedicine Association has a website with links to various organizations and its recommendations regarding telemedicine. Go to *www.atmeda.org* to learn more. (For a bonus checklist on bylaws and this chapter's standards, see Figure 3.17.)

3.17	Chart for Review of Bylaws for Compliance with TJC Standards Required Documentation

Required Element	Current Location	Proposed Location in Bylaws and Comments
MS.01.01.01 Medical staff self-governance and accountability		
EP 8 Bylaws state that the office of the medical staff can adopt and amend MS bylaws, R&R, and policies, and can propose these directly to the governing body		
EP 9 The medical staff may choose to delegate authority to make proposals for changes in rules, regulations, or policies to the medical executive committee (MEC). This EP applies if the OMS has delegated this authority to the MEC and the governing body has approved the delegation.		
EP 10 The medical staff must have a process to manage any conflicts that may arise between the medical staff and the MEC regarding recommendations to adopt or change rules, regulations, or policies and other issues that may occur. Using a mechanism determined by the governing body, medical staff members may communicate to the governing body regarding a rule, regulation, or policy adopted by the MEC or by the OMS.		Although this is not required by TJC to be in the bylaws, the bylaws may be a good place to include this mechanism.

3.17	Chart for Review of Bylaws for Compliance with TJC Standards Required Documentation *(cont.)*	

Required Element	Current Location	Proposed Location in Bylaws and Comments
EP 11 There may be an incident in which a critical change to rules and regulations may be necessary in order to comply with law or regulation. In these cases, there can be a process for the MEC to provisionally adopt and the board to provisionally approve these amendments without notifying the medical staff. This authority must be delegated by the voting members of the OMS. If this urgent amendment is required, the MEC must immediately notify the medical staff of the change and the medical staff must be given the opportunity for retrospective review and comment. If the medical staff and MEC are in agreement, the amendment stands, but if there is a disagreement, the conflict resolution process is implemented.		
EP 12 Medical staff structure		
EP 13 Qualifications for appointment to the OMS		
EP 14 Credentialing/recredentialing and privileging/ reprivileging process for LIPs and other practitioners and the process for appointment and reappointment to membership on the medical staff		
EP 15 The duties and privileges for each medical staff category of the medical staff (e.g., active, courtesy)		

3.17 Chart for Review of Bylaws for Compliance with TJC Standards Required Documentation *(cont.)*

Required Element	Current Location	Proposed Location in Bylaws and Comments
EP 16 Requirements for completing and documenting H&Ps. Check to make sure that bylaws include a requirement that the patient receives the H&P no more than 30 days prior to, or within 24 hours after registration or inpatient admission, and prior to surgery or a procedure requiring anesthesia. Also check to make sure that for an H&P that was completed within 30 days prior to registration or inpatient admission, an update documenting any changes in the patient's condition is required to be completed within 24 hours after registration or inpatient admission, and prior to surgery or a procedure requiring anesthesia.		
EP 17 Description of MS members authorized to vote		
EP 18 Process for selection, election, and removal of medical staff officers		
EP 19 Medical staff officer positions		
EP 20 Function, size, and composition of the MEC. If authority is delegated to the MEC to act on behalf of the medical staff, such authority is documented, as is the mechanism for delegation or removal of this authority.		
EP 21 Process for selecting, electing, and removing MEC members		
EP 22 Documentation that the MEC includes physicians and may include others if established by the OMS		

3.17   Chart for Review of Bylaws for Compliance with TJC Standards Required Documentation *(cont.)*

Required Element	Current Location	Proposed Location in Bylaws and Comments
EP 23 Documentation that the MEC has authority to act on behalf of the medical staff between meetings is included in the defined responsibilities of the MEC		
EP 24 Process for adopting and amending MS bylaws		
EP 25 Process for adopting and amending MS rules & regulations, and policies		
EP 26 Process for credentialing/recredentialing and privileging/reprivileging LIPs and other practitioners		
EP 27 Process for MS appointment and reappointment		
EP 28 Indications for automatic suspension of MS membership or clinical privileges		
EP 29 Indications for summary suspension of medical staff membership or clinical privileges		
EP 30 Indications for recommending termination or suspension of medical staff membership, and/or termination, suspension, or reduction of clinical privileges		
EP 31 Process for automatic suspension and summary suspension of MS membership or clinical privileges		
EP 32 Process for summary suspension of MS membership or clinical privileges		
EP 33 Process for recommending termination or suspension of MS membership and/or termination, suspension, or reduction of clinical privileges		

3.17 Chart for Review of Bylaws for Compliance with TJC Standards Required Documentation *(cont.)*

Required Element	Current Location	Proposed Location in Bylaws and Comments
EP 34 Process for fair hearing and appeal of an adverse recommendation, including how hearings and appeals are scheduled and conducted and the composition of the hearing committee		
EP 35 Composition of hearing committee		
EP 36 When departments of the OMS exist, the qualifications and roles and responsibilities of the department chair, including the following:		
Appropriate board certification or comparable competence established through credentialing process		
Clinically related activities		
Administratively related activities (not required if services provided by the hospital)		
Continuing observation of the professional performance of individuals in department with delineated clinical privileges		
Recommending criteria to the MS for clinical privileges relevant to the care provided in the department		
Recommending clinical privileges for department members		
Assessing and recommending off-site sources for needed services not provided by the department or the organization		

| 3.17 | Chart for Review of Bylaws for Compliance with TJC Standards Required Documentation *(cont.)* | | |

Required Element	Current Location	Proposed Location in Bylaws and Comments
The integration of the department or service into the primary functions of the organization and coordination and integration of interdepartmental and intradepartmental services		
Developing and implementing policies and procedures that guide the department and support the provision of care, treatment, and services		
Recommending an adequate number of qualified and competent persons to provide care, treatment, and services		
Determining qualifications and competency for non-LIP departmental personnel providing patient care, treatment, or services		
Ongoing assessment and improvement of the quality of patient care, treatment, and services		
Maintaining quality control programs		
Orienting and providing continuing education to all persons in the department or service		
Recommending space and other needed departmental resources		
MS.02.01.01 Medical Executive Committee		
EP 1 The structure and function of the MEC conforms to the MS bylaws		

3.17	**Chart for Review of Bylaws for Compliance with TJC Standards Required Documentation** *(cont.)*	
EP 3 All MS members are eligible for MEC membership		
EP 6 MEC has a mechanism to recommend MS termination		
EP 8 MEC makes MS membership recommendations directly to the governing body as defined in the bylaws		
EP 9 MEC makes recommendations about the MS structure directly to the governing body as defined in the bylaws		
EP 10 MEC makes recommendations regarding the process used to review credentials and delineate privileges directly to the governing body as defined in the bylaws		
EP 11 MEC makes recommendations regarding privileges delineation directly to the governing body as defined in the bylaws		
EP 12 MEC makes recommendations to the governing body regarding the MEC's authority to review and act on the reports of medical staff committees, departments, and other groups or committees who are assigned a specific function as defined in the bylaws.		
MS.06.01.05 Privileging		
EP 11 Completed privileging applications must be within the specified time period specified in the bylaws		